## Wyggeston and Queen Elizabeth I College

Please return the book on or before t

KT-431-753

16. JUN. 1998

11 JAN

...known for his work on behalf
. He has life-long experience of
...ilies whose lives have been shattered
by unpleasant and unwelcome change. His approach to
cancer in this book is strongly influenced by his
professional knowledge and expertise, and by his
personal experience of trying to understand and come to
terms with the impact of cancer within his own family.
He is also the author of *Coping Successfully with Pain*
(Sheldon Press, 1992).

Wyggeston QE I

00228195

# Overcoming Common Problems Series

For a full list of titles please contact
Sheldon Press, Marylebone Road, London NW1 4DU

**The Assertiveness Workbook**
A plan for busy women
JOANNA GUTMANN

**Birth Over Thirty**
SHEILA KITZINGER

**Body Language**
How to read others' thoughts by their
gestures
ALLAN PEASE

**Body Language in Relationships**
DAVID COHEN

**Calm Down**
How to cope with frustration and anger
DR PAUL HAUCK

**Changing Course**
How to take charge of your career
SUE DYSON AND STEPHEN HOARE

**Comfort for Depression**
JANET HORWOOD

**Coping Successfully with Agoraphobia**
DR KENNETH HAMBLY

**Coping Successfully with Migraine**
SUE DYSON

**Coping Successfully with Pain**
NEVILLE SHONE

**Coping Successfully with Panic Attacks**
SHIRLEY TRICKETT

**Coping Successfully with Prostate Problems**
ROSY REYNOLDS

**Coping Successfully with Your Hyperactive Child**
DR PAUL CARSON

**Coping Successfully with Your Irritable Bowel**
ROSEMARY NICOL

**Coping Successfully with Your Second Child**
FIONA MARSHALL

**Coping with Anxiety and Depression**
SHIRLEY TRICKETT

**Coping with Blushing**
DR ROBERT EDELMANN

**Coping with Cot Death**
SARAH MURPHY

**Coping with Depression and Elation**
DR PATRICK McKEON

**Coping with Strokes**
DR TOM SMITH

**Coping with Suicide**
DR DONALD SCOTT

**Coping with Thrush**
CAROLINE CLAYTON

**Curing Arthritis Diet Book**
MARGARET HILLS

**Curing Arthritis – The Drug-Free Way**
MARGARET HILLS

**Curing Arthritis**
More ways to a drug-free life
MARGARET HILLS

**Curing Coughs, Colds and Flu – The Drug-Free Way**
MARGARET HILLS

**Curing Illness – The Drug-Free Way**
MARGARET HILLS

**Depression**
DR PAUL HAUCK

**Divorce and Separation**
Every woman's guide to a new life
ANGELA WILLANS

**Don't Blame Me!**
How to stop blaming yourself
and other people
TONY GOUGH

**Everything You Need to Know about Shingles**
DR ROBERT YOUNGSON

**Family First Aid and Emergency Handbook**
DR ANDREW STANWAY

# Overcoming Common Problems Series

# Overcoming Common Problems Series

**Overcoming Common Problems**

# CANCER
# – A FAMILY AFFAIR

## Neville Shone

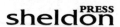

First published in Great Britain in 1995 by
Sheldon Press, SPCK, Marylebone Road, London NW1 4DU

© Neville Shone 1995

All rights reserved. No part of this book may be reproduced
or transmitted in any form or by any means, electronic or
mechanical, including photocopying, recording, or by any
information storage and retrieval system, without permission
in writing from the publisher.

Acc. No.

00228195

Class No.
616 · 99 SHO

British Library Cataloguing-in-Publication Data
A catalogue record for this book is available from the British Library

ISBN 0–85969–706–1

Photoset by Deltatype Ltd, Ellesmere Port, Cheshire
Printed in Great Britain by Biddles Ltd, Guildford and King's Lynn

# Contents

Wyggeston QEI College
Library

# Acknowledgements

This book could not have been written without the valuable help, information, advice, and support from the following:

People with first-hand experience of cancer, as patients, as relatives, and as parents of children with the disease, who willingly gave me their time and talked to me of their experiences in the hope that they would help those being faced with the illness for the first time. I am deeply grateful to them for their help, and their willingness to share what must have been, for many of them, very painful memories.

Pain Association Scotland (formerly PLUS) for constant support and assistance, for organizing contact with some of their members, their families, group organizers, and counsellors, and for putting their library at my disposal to assist my research.

Sister Jeanette Bain, for giving me insight into her work as a Macmillan nurse in Dumfries and Galloway.

POSY, Yorkhill Hospital, Glasgow. These parents of children with cancer provided a most useful insight into their problems.

Ann Robarts, medical social worker, Arrowepark Hospital, Birkenhead, Merseyside, for her invaluable contribution concerning her professional work with children and their families and the work of CHICS (a children's cancer support group in her area).

BACUP, CancerLink, and Cancer Relief Macmillan Fund for providing a wide selection of leaflets detailing information about their work and service to people with cancer and their families.

The names and other identifying facts contained in the case histories used in this book have been changed in order to protect the privacy of those concerned. These alterations in no way influence the value of the examples.

*Neville Shone*
*Arbroath*
*July 1994*

# Introduction

Cancer is a family affair that has a profound influence on the lives of every member of the families concerned. Most books written on cancer present a very clear understanding of its causes and progression, and provide a wealth of detail on specific manifestations of the illness. Thus it is not my intention to repeat what has already been well recorded elsewhere. Rather, I want to go on from there and ask what can be done to help the patient and members of the family to come to terms and cope with the illness and the impact it has on their lives.

All serious illness brings unavoidable practical and emotional adjustments, and out of necessity forces family members to make temporary changes to their way of life. On the whole, after a period of a few weeks, as the crisis subsides, life returns to normal. Cancer, however, is marked by the fact that it is immediately identified in people's minds as being life-threatening, uncertain in its outcome, and prolonged. It may be punctuated by many periods of acute anxiety about the patient's well-being. Each such period is unsettling in itself, but because the outcome is uncertain – even during periods of long remission – there is the ever-present fear that the illness might recur. There is no time for anyone to sit back, breathe a sigh of relief, and comfortably return to the pre-illness status quo.

At first, practical adjustments will seem to take place automatically. They may not be ideal, but the family will manage and in the short term the arrangements will be adequate. However, the emotional adjustments are not so easy. Fear and anxiety in the patient and other family members may prevail and be fuelled at frequent intervals during the course of the illness. There is nothing like fear and anxiety for wasting energy that could be used in the healing process. Both fear and anxiety limit our capacity to cope.

In many ways, cancer is similar to all chronic illness and other long-term crises that affect the family: it provokes strong feelings, challenges the strength of existing relationships, and forces people to take on burdens that they have never carried before. They may rise to the challenge and emerge stronger than ever, or they may find everything just too much for them. People will react in many different ways. The family affected by cancer will have its own

1

pattern of living, its own system of relationships and ways of ordering things that have ensured that, up to the point of diagnosis, people's needs have been met in a more or less satisfactory way – in other words, a reasonable degree of harmony has probably been reached between the members that has enabled them to cope with day-to-day activities. Yet the family is always in a state of change as people pass through the various stages of development from childhood to old age. These changes are accepted as being normal and, although they bring their stresses, most families are able to absorb them and come to terms with them. Such stresses include getting married, pregnancy and childbirth, a child's first day at school, starting work or changing a job, someone leaving home, moving house, separation, divorce, or perhaps the death of a partner or parent. All these changes create anxieties that are potentially destructive to each and every member of the family, but they are events to which people usually adapt. They are part of life, and each of these experiences influences the way we relate to others and cope with subsequent crises. We may not come through such events unscathed, but for the most part we are able to put them in some sort of perspective. They may make us fearful and defensive, but they are not necessarily so destructive that they prevent us from taking on new challenges and attempting to live life to the full.

The family may be likened to a container in which the members move around each other, each living individual lives that constantly impinge on the lives of the others. The link in a family is emotional. Even though in some cases people may not be very close, and may even be physically separated, they have shared memories of good and bad experiences, shared disappointments, suffering and loss, and perhaps even the memory of conflict. The feelings generated within families are very strong, but they are not always feelings of love and affection. Anger and guilt can be experienced in the family more strongly than in any other situation. At its best, the family might be likened to a spider's web – strong, yet delicately balanced, and where any pressure on one part will trigger the other parts to take up the additional strain and provide support. Sometimes the adjustment is successful; at other times, damage may result, and time will be needed to make repairs.

A diagnosis of cancer in one member of the family immediately threatens all members of that family. It is a disease that produces negative images and fears for each family member. Anxieties generated within the 'container' of the family bounce from one person to another, establishing an emotional climate that is as potentially destructive as the disease itself.

This book aims to help people understand these strong forces and to suggest ways of limiting the destruction. Whether you go through the experience of cancer as a patient or as a relative of the patient, I want to reassure you that you can come through the experience. Whatever the outcome, the experience has the potential to enrich and strengthen you, even though you may bear the scars of battle.

Very few families are untouched by cancer. It is a fact of life that most adults will have the experience of a number of relatives and close friends living – and dying – with cancer. This book has emerged from reflection on my own experiences. My earliest such experience was at the age of five, and today, some 50 years later, I am really only now fully appreciating the impact that the cancer suffered by my father (and his subsequent death) had on my mother and myself, grandparents, uncles, and aunts. Early events are thrown into relief by subsequent experiences, and we often discover that we have learned useful lessons that stand us in good stead in facing new challenges. However, later experiences with cancer have found me just as unprepared as I had been the first time. I suppose this happens with most severe crises, but there seems to be something about the intensity of the impact of the news of this particular illness that obliterates all our previous learning about how to cope. We experience each particular occurrence as unique. We have to go through every stage of adjustment and experience every feeling as though for the first time. Yet this is not quite true, for we find ourselves remembering vividly all the emotional pain of previous experiences, and this in itself adds to the present crisis.

When my first wife was diagnosed as suffering from cancer, the shock was so great that it felt as though a wall had been erected between her and the rest of the family. It seemed that with this diagnosis, a close family member had left, and been replaced by another person occupying the same physical body; someone we had to get to know afresh. At this time I was not aware that this is a common phenomenon: that when someone is seriously ill and frightened, their attention is focused within themselves – controlling the fear, controlling the panic – such that their ability to respond normally to others is extremely limited. I was only vaguely aware that I too, along with my children, was absorbed in my own inner turmoil, facing up to the fear of the unknown and an unpredictable future, coping with the fact that life as we had known it was over.

At the time, we knew so little about cancer and its treatment. Like many others, I saw the aims of treatment as being entirely directed towards a cure, and when this did not happen in a matter of weeks, we all shared the experience of failure – and this at a time when it seemed as if we were completely exhausted, and with little left in reserve to face the next stage – whatever it might be.

None of us was prepared for the physical and psychological impact of the treatment, and were confused by some of the discomfort, wondering whether it resulted from the illness itself or whether it was a side-effect of the treatment. Should we call the doctor? Should we wait and see if it eases? It all seemed such a muddle. We did not always know the right questions, or who to ask. Neither were we aware of the outside support system and how to go about getting it. Even if we had known, the emotional impact of the whole experience drained our energy, inhibited action, and made us feel isolated and negative. No matter how good you may be at work, as an administrator, organizer, manager, teacher, etc., a diagnosis of cancer may make you feel helpless and totally inadequate.

As in my own family's experience, many people are completely unprepared and muddle through, learning from experience at a time when they are in a state of shock, extreme anxiety, beset with fears about cancer, forms of treatment, and long-term prospects. This book is directed towards people diagnosed as having cancer, carers, family, and friends. Its primary aim is to provide an understanding of the emotional impact of the illness, and to build on this understanding in order to cope more effectively.

Because of a lack of clarity about what the professionals are trying to do to help, there is often confusion and anger in the patient and the family; this uses up valuable energy that can be better directed towards healing and coping with the illness. It is hoped that the following pages will make it easier for the patient, family, and carers to understand and communicate realistically with the professionals, and also between themselves.

My purpose in this book is to:

- make available knowledge about cancer and its causes, and the various forms of treatment and their side-effects;
- highlight valuable methods of coping;
- identify available support services;
- help bring about an understanding of what the professionals are trying to do to help;

- remove any idea that the illness is a punishment or the result of some kind of defect in the personality of the individual. Lack of understanding in this area often causes confusion and anger in the patient and family.

By focusing on the emotional aspects of the illness, it is hoped that it will be easier for all concerned to understand and to communicate effectively with professionals, and with other members of the family.

Many people have contributed to this book by giving me the benefit of their experience of having cancer, or caring for someone in the family during their illness. All of those interviewed focused on the emotional burden they carried during the course of the illness, and in the periods of adjustment afterwards. They all stressed that they had somehow become 'experts' in medical terminology, who were quite able to swap big words with one another, but they all felt that information by itself did nothing to help them cope with the sense of isolation, fear, threat of loss, and confusion that they frequently experienced. These feelings were there, but had not been voiced – even within their own family circle.

My own experience of cancer in the family, further informed by the experience of the many people I interviewed (patients, family members, doctors, social workers, nurses, and charity workers), has added greatly to my understanding of the impact of the illness. As I read the literature on the subject and reflected on the experience of others, I could not help but relate my thinking to my own experience of serious painful illness, which led me to write *Coping Successfully with Pain*. I have experienced despair, fear, and helplessness – conditions severe enough in themselves to merit specialized attention. I have experienced the psychological barriers that exist between the ill person and all others who are involved. I have felt the strong waves of apprehension coming from each member of my family, which added still further to my isolation. I have experienced the feeling of being worthless; frightened that I would never regain any degree of independence. I lived for a long time with the feeling that decisions about me were being made by other people, and that everyone else shared a secret that I knew nothing about. I lost confidence in the ability of doctors and hospitals to offer any kind of help. To all intents and purposes, I suffered a death of the spirit. You will probably recognize your own feelings, but I want to reassure you that the spirit is in fact very strong and, despite the ravages of cancer, will eventually survive and be strengthened.

You may have picked up this book because you or someone close to you has just been diagnosed as having cancer. Or it may be because you, or they, have not been diagnosed yet, but have discovered some abnormality that is causing concern. You may have already started on a process of investigation, or you may be too frightened to embark on this process – fearing that it will confirm your worst fears. The greatest fear is of the unknown, and this book sets out to inform, guide, and comfort anyone who has cancer, or is involved in the care of someone with the illness – either a family member or close friend. It will be valuable reading at any stage in the illness – for carers, for families, for counsellors, or anyone with an interest in the subject. It may be particularly useful for those who have been through the experience, and now want to make sense of, and come to terms with, what has happened to them and their loved ones.

Over the years I have struggled to make sense of the whole experience of severe chronic illness, and to relate this to my previous work as a social worker with families, and as a teacher concerned to convey knowledge and professional standards to emerging social workers. This book is the result of my struggle.

# 1

# Understanding Cancer

There have been many books, magazine articles, and television programmes on the subject of cancer over the last 15 years or so, all of which have provided invaluable information about the nature of the disease and the various treatments available; and at some time or other most of us have donated money, time, or energy to cancer research and related care projects. Yet if we are told we have cancer, or someone close to us is diagnosed as having the illness, we often discover that we possess very little real knowledge. It seems that understanding and learning often only take place when there is an overwhelming motivation to find out, and it is usually the proximity of the illness that provides this motivation. In spite of this strong motivation, it takes time to learn about cancer and understand the available treatments, side-effects, and strategies for coping. Unfortunately, the nature of the cancer, and the medical processes that are triggered off by the diagnosis, do not allow us the luxury of the necessary time for this learning process. In practice, we have to learn as we go along, and we find ourselves already in the crisis before we are intellectually and emotionally prepared for it.

We have all had the experience, perhaps when talking to an electrician, a plumber, computer expert, or a car mechanic, of being completely ignorant of the explanations they are giving us for the problems we might be facing in our domestic lives. Usually, we are not really interested in the details – we just want to know how quickly the fault can be put right. To some extent, this is how we are when faced with the medical expert who tells us we have an illness. Our bodies have 'broken down', and we expect him to put things right. It is often the lack of knowledge and understanding of even the basics that is at the root of many of the communication problems that exist between doctors and patients. In this situation it is the expert, the person who has the knowledge, who also has the power. When you are short of knowledge, there is very little that you can do to argue your case. If it is you that has been diagnosed as having cancer, you may sense that a course of action is not suitable for you, but you are powerless because you have no grounds on which to dispute it. Therefore you can easily feel you have no control over decisions about the kind of treatment proposed for you. This often leads to a passivity throughout the whole family, which results in total surrender to the efforts of the professionals and the feeling that there is nothing we can do for ourselves that can influence the course of the illness.

In this chapter I shall try to provide information to help you develop your own understanding of cancer and its treatment. Possessing this basic information won't make you an expert, but it will help to create a sense of involvement in the treatment process and to develop a sense of partnership with the professionals. The more active your participation, the less likely it is that you will feel you have lost control over your own life. You will be more able to understand the reasons behind the decisions your doctor may wish to take, and feel more confident about the questions to ask and, perhaps, even to suggest alternative approaches. This confidence is important for the whole family as they support one another through a difficult time.

Perhaps more importantly, having this knowledge will help you to control your fear, for fear and ignorance are closely related.

## What is cancer?

Cancer is a disease of the cells. Cells are the smallest building blocks in our bodies, and can only be seen under a microscope. Every part of the human body is made up of many thousands of cells, which combine to form many different types of tissue – muscle, skin, bone, blood, glands, and other organs.

Tissue is made up of specialized cells that perform specific functions. Within each cell is a central control (or nucleus) that contains chromosomes. Each chromosome is the home of many thousands of genes that are made up of DNA, which controls the cell's activities.

Cells normally reproduce themselves in order to replace those that have become damaged or died, or if more cells are needed for some special reason. Some cells, like those for making blood, are replaced more often than others. It may surprise you to know that white blood cells are completely replaced every six hours, and this rate of reproduction is increased during infection when more are needed. Cells reproduce by division; each cell splits in half to produce a 'daughter' cell, thus making an exact copy of itself in order to continue performing whatever functions it is programmed to perform. This constant renewal ensures that the tissues of the body remain healthy and in good repair. Cells divide according to commands from the genetic material (DNA) at the centre of each cell.

Sometimes, it seems, the genes controlling growth and development become overactive and send out too many signals. The cell responds by dividing again and again, far beyond the normal needs of the body. This uncontrollable growth of cells may cause a swelling or tumour, which indicates that it is likely they have encroached on to neighbouring tissue or dispersed into the bloodstream. These cells do not obey the various commands of the body. Reproducing wildly, they renew themselves more often than the normal cells surrounding them, and, what is more, they do not perform any useful function for the good of the body.

## Types of tumour

Tumours may be benign or malignant, but most tumours are benign. They are called benign because they cannot spread to other parts of the body. They are generally called fibromas, adenomas, neoplasms, or simply benign tumours. If they grow too large they may damage vital organs, and because of this risk they will probably need to be removed surgically to eliminate the problem once and for all. It is important, therefore, that lumps of any kind should be investigated. They should *never* be ignored.

When we talk of cancer we are talking of a malignant growth or tumour. A malignant tumour can also sometimes be referred to as a carcinoma, sarcoma, or blastoma, depending on the type of tissue from which it has arisen.

Cancers, or malignant tumours, have two special features:

- they can spread to nearby organs or tissues;
- cancer cells can break off from the original tumour, and may be carried in the bloodstream to distant sites in the body where they may form new tumours called 'metastases' or 'secondaries'.

It is because cancer cells can spread to vital organs (such as the lungs or liver) and affect their normal function that cancer anywhere in the body is a potentially life-threatening disease. Cancer in its earliest stage, i.e. its pre-invasive stage, is still localized and highly curable. If not caught at this stage and left untreated, the cancer begins to invade the surrounding tissue.

Although at this point it is still 'localized' and has not spread to other areas of the body, once it has invaded the surrounding tissue then the cancer can be considered to have reached a serious stage. The tumour may become so large that it crowds out healthy cells, destroying them and reducing their ability to function. It may be that the tumour forms an obstruction, or exerts dangerous pressure on nearby vital organs. Surgical treatment at this stage can still produce a cure, though the parts of the body being invaded may also need to be removed.

Cancers vary in their ability to spread. Some start to move to another site in the body quite quickly, whereas others take longer. It is interesting to note that this spread conforms to a pattern. For example, bowel tumours have a tendency to spread to the liver, while breast cancers spread to the bones, and lung tumours to the brain. In general, the longer a tumour exists, the greater the likelihood that it has shed cells that progress to different parts of the body via the bloodstream or lymphatic system.

The lymphatic system is the body's natural drainage system, a series of ducts that carry away excess fluid. The doctor will examine specific points in the neck, chest, under the arms, the groin, and the abdomen where there are collecting points known as lymph nodes, to see whether a cancer has spread. A swelling at one of these points may be the first indication to a person that they have cancer. As lumps can form in these areas for other reasons, it is important that any changes in these areas are reported to a doctor. More likely than not, these lumps will be harmless and your doctor will be able to reassure you.

The lymphatic system is an important part of the body's defence against all manner of disease. It is a vital part of our immune system, which is thought to be as important in defending against cancer as it is against bacteria or viruses. It may even be that cancer cells are controlled by the immune system in their early stages before they reproduce sufficiently to build up a cancer large enough to be detected.

There is good evidence to suggest that the immune system can be weakened because of age, stress, environmental factors, nutritional deficiencies, or simply heredity. Overwhelming infection can also weaken the immune system, and a weakened system is unable to destroy the abnormal cells.

Cancer cells have their own built-in defence system, which enables them to produce a protective coating that is not recognized by the immune system – thus enabling them to slip by undetected.

Current research is directed towards producing new drugs to strengthen the immune system. Anyone with cancer can do much to bolster the effectiveness of their immune system by ensuring that their general health is maintained, stress is reduced and controlled, and a healthy diet adopted.

It is ironic that the three major forms of treatment for cancer, i.e. surgery, radiation, and chemotherapy, all have the effect of weakening the immune system. Because of this, a lot of attention is paid to ensuring that anyone undergoing these treatments maintains a high level of nutrition. Frequent examinations of the blood are made to assess the impact of the treatment on the red and white blood cells. The white blood cells, in particular, play a crucial part in maintaining the health of the immune system.

Although the majority of cancers are solid tumours – i.e. large lumps of cells, more often than not occurring in the lungs, bowel, or breast – there are others that are cancers of the blood, generally known as leukaemia. In this case, the body produces large numbers of abnormal cells that move around in the bloodstream and attack the healthy blood cells.

## Common forms of cancer

There is a tendency among lay people when they hear the word 'cancer' to assume that it is one disease, and that every cancer behaves in the same way. However, this is not so. Cancer is a blanket expression for more than two hundred separate forms of the illness. So, just as there is no single type of cancer, there cannot possibly be a single cause, nor is it possible to say that all cases of any one type are caused by the same factors.

Cancer can attack any part of the body, but lung, breast, and bowel cancers are the most common forms in the Western world. Perhaps rarest are tumours of the bones and the body's connective tissues.

Cancer is most common in old age, which is not altogether surprising since those in developed countries are living longer as a result of the success in controlling most of the infectious diseases that once killed many people in childhood or early adulthood. Cancer may even be part of the natural process of the body 'closing down' and losing its ability to carry out its normal repair functions and to fight disease. Cancer is very rare in children and young people, and when they do contract it they are more likely to have leukaemia and cancer of the lymph glands, bone, or nerve cancers.

## *What are the causes?*

When we come to consider the causes of cancer, we enter something of a minefield. Examination of research suggests that cancer can be associated with

- heredity
- lifestyle
- environment
- chance

No one knows exactly what are the 'right' conditions to trigger the process of a cell getting out of control. It is well known that you are more likely to get cancer if you are exposed to such things as radiation, asbestos, or cigarette-smoking. In fact, smoking is responsible for almost one-third of all cancer deaths in the UK. However, not every smoker will develop cancer. Likewise, people who have never smoked may develop lung cancer through passive smoking, i.e. constantly being in the company of those who are smoking.

Some people are more susceptible to cancer as a result of hereditary factors, but only if they are exposed to other factors that are capable of triggering the disease. Paradoxically, people with no sign that they have an inherited susceptibility may still develop cancer.

Some research has suggested links between individual personality, emotional attitudes, and vulnerability to cancer, but at this stage it would be wrong to suggest that these factors have any proven link with causation. One of the problems in the way that this research has been reported over the last few years is that it has led to people feeling that it is some 'fault' within themselves that has given rise to cancer. When this happens, it is but a small step for those with the illness to feel they are weak or are being punished. They may develop feelings of guilt for something that is entirely beyond their control. So, if you have the disease and someone is telling you that your personality needs to be completely restructured, then show them the door! However, it may be the case, when the initial stages of the illness have been dealt with and you have entered remission, that you need to think about making some changes in your lifestyle that will enable you to enjoy a full and balanced life. Anyone who has had a serious illness needs to think about adjusting certain aspects of their lives to limit the demands made on them, and to reduce stress. They may need to think about pacing themselves, with a better balance between work and leisure. It may even be that they have to be more aware of their own needs.

Stress has also been suggested as a trigger for a person developing cancer, but there are problems in defining what stress actually is and why some people thrive on stress while it makes others ill. Stressful life events such as bereavement or divorce are also difficult to pinpoint as triggers, because the time between cells beginning to turn cancerous and the point at which symptoms are evident may be months or even years.

Diet has also been suggested as a possible causative factor, particularly as countries with a higher standard of living have a higher rate of deaths from bowel and stomach cancers. It has been pointed out that in the Western world we tend to eat rich, refined foods, while diets in poorer countries are higher in fibre and lower in protein. Another possibility is that the food-refining process exposes us to possible cancer-causing agents. As yet, though, no one has been able to identify these cancer-causing agents. Furthermore, there is no evidence to suggest that any of the chemicals used in food preservation can, by themselves, cause cancer. (At the same time, there is no scientific proof that they are harmless either!)

Much has been done during the last century to cut down the risk of exposure to known cancer-causing (carcinogenic) pollutants within the workplace – for example, asbestos; and Health and Safety regulations have rigid requirements for the handling of any carcinogenic substances. However, no one knows how many people get cancer as a result of environmental pollution. It is my own opinion that while there is any doubt at all, the whole of Western society should think very seriously about the known amount of pollution, cancer-causing or not. Whatever else pollution does, it makes life very unpleasant, and there is evidence that people living in polluted areas have more illness generally than the rest of the population. As a nation we seem to have become too tolerant of the pollution of the environment caused by industry and traffic. We all know that certain areas of the country carry a yellow/grey 'umbrella', and I for one know that at the end of a long journey on a traffic-choked motorway I feel extreme discomfort around the eyes and in my respiratory system. Continued exposure to such conditions is not to be recommended.

Recent research has indicated that a susceptibility to certain cancers – including breast, ovarian, and bowel cancer – could be passed on in the genes. If the susceptibility is inherited, it does not automatically follow that cancer will manifest itself in brothers and sisters or in subsequent generations. Other factors seem to be responsible for triggering the illness. The risk of developing inherited cancers is found to be only marginally greater than the overall risk to the general population. The positive result of isolating genes responsible for the transmission of cancer means that it will be possible to screen and monitor any family members who might be at risk, thus allowing for early detection and treatment.

So as far as causes are concerned, for every theory there is a counter-theory, and the honest answer is that there is a lot we still don't know. This last section about causation has been included specifically to underline the fact that if you have the illness yourself, or a member of your family has it, it is pointless spending time and energy speculating on what you or they might or might not have done to have caused the disease. All available energy is needed to get well.

# 2

## Hearing the News
## and Goals of Treatment

Many people on hearing the news that they have cancer immediately translate the doctor's words as a message that they are going to die. It is for this reason that people with a diagnosis of cancer need time – time to reflect alone, and with those closest to them, time to be heard, time to have things explained, time to be reassured. Thus the person who conveys the news should take the time to instil hope for recovery.

### *Breaking the news gently*

Unfortunately, people are often given the news of their illness, and then, while still in shock and possibly paralysed with fear, they are asked to carry on a discussion about proposed forms of treatment. After such traumatic news, it is little wonder that they are dumbstruck. All too frequently the doctor may ask, 'Have you any questions?', and overawed at hearing a diagnosis of cancer shock and fear can paralyse the intellect, slow down the thinking process, and cause a whole welter of thoughts and anxieties about the future to crowd in, producing a state of utter confusion. You will need time to take in what you have been told and to regain enough stability to be able to make decisions. You may even need someone else to sit down quietly with you and go over the news once again, and be ready to discuss its implications at a pace you can cope with.

This is no time to be involved in making decisions about treatment that may be life-saving, but have major repercussions on your future quality of life. With the exception of a few very fast-growing cancers, some days – or even a week or two – will not make the difference between life and death. It is important, therefore, wherever possible, for doctor and patient to pause for thought, allowing time for discussion with other members of the family, and for assessment of the kind of help that will be necessary during the illness. The breathing space is also a time to collect information about the illness and the various forms of treatment available.

Knowledge and being appropriately informed is essential to the coping process. Fear of the unknown debilitates, depresses, and reduces a person's capacity to cope with all aspects of illness. Ignorance leads not only to fear, but to fantasies about the disease that in turn produce even more fear. Appropriate information can help put fears and anxieties into perspective. Ideally, your medical advisers should be the source of this information.

Evidence suggests that all too often the medical profession underestimate patients' needs for knowledge about their particular disease and its treatment. If you have been told you have cancer, the question of how much information is necessary is the joint responsibility of you and your doctor. It is up to the professionals to recognize and be sensitive to the traumatic impact of the diagnosis and to anticipate that shock may impede your ability to take in the news. Patients and their families can be helped considerably by having available information booklets, tapes, and/or videos. This information needs to be accompanied by face-to-face contact, providing space for discussion and questions.

However, professional communicators often assume that if they have provided information, the listener hears it and takes it in. They forget that the listener may be so busy digesting part of the message, or responding internally on an emotional level, that everything else is simply driven from their mind. Hence many questions are left unasked. Also, patients may refrain from questioning because they have already anticipated the possible answers, and would rather not have their worst fears confirmed. The professional therefore has a responsibility to anticipate what these 'taboo' topics might be and open them up for discussion.

## A sensitive diagnostic service

It will be apparent from this that I am advocating a sophisticated diagnostic service that goes beyond the basic provision of information about the illness, its treatment, side-effects, and possible outcome. This kind of service should not be seen as a luxury available only under private medicine, but should be given as a right to all patients and their families simply because they are human beings. It means accepting that the thinking, feeling, and spiritual qualities of people are every bit as important as their physical bodies. It also means recognizing that technically competent medical staff may not always be fitted by temperament or training to carry out this delicate work. I do not intend this to be a criticism of the work of people in the medical services, but merely to point out that technical competence, medical training, and the service generally provided is not enough. These comments apply not just to cancer, but to any anxiety-provoking situation that brings someone within the scope of the medical services. Communication needs to go beyond the surface 'How may I help you?' and 'Have a nice day!' level, which often seems to be a substitute for real communication and caring.

It must be acknowledged that patients carry a multiple burden when attending hospital. Not only are they overwhelmed by thoughts of what may be wrong with them, but they may feel shy or intimidated by the whole experience of the hospital building, the uniforms, the formality, administrative procedures, meeting a succession of strangers, and working out where they fit in with their problem.

There was one common factor which linked most of those I interviewed in the course of my research; it was the feeling that they had been treated with a lack of sensitivity during their early encounters with hospital staff. When anyone seeks medical treatment they are likely to feel very fragile, vulnerable, and low in morale. Anything said to you at this time is likely to have a very strong emotional impact, so it is quite easy to see how people can perceive sometimes quite ordinary business-like treatment as 'insensitive'. All people interviewed felt that their perceived lack of sensitivity damaged their trust in those professionals responsible for their care. If you feel you have been treated with a lack of sensitivity it is important that your feelings are not allowed to become so obsessive that they waste the energy needed to fight the illness. Strong feelings of this kind can interfere with your ability to establish a sense of partnership with the professionals. It is important if you feel this way to talk to a counsellor or social worker to get your feelings off your chest, get them into perspective, and help in your preparation to cope with whatever lies ahead.

When you are confronted with a medical consultation you may not want to appear ignorant by asking what might seem a foolish question. Remember, *no* question is foolish, and no question is too basic if it is about something you do not understand. You may feel that questions waste the time of a 'busy' doctor, and some doctors can give this impression – knowingly or unknowingly. These factors reinforce your feelings of being powerless, especially when doctors seem to be able to decide your fate, to give or withhold treatment, to relieve pain.

It is important for your own peace of mind, if for no other reason, to be able to raise questions or voice your fears – if not actually to your doctor, then to someone you trust: a relative, friend, or another professional. Sometimes trust comes only after you have taken the risk and faced up to a fear by sharing it with someone else.

## Thinking about treatment

No matter how well the information about the diagnosis is given and no matter how much consideration is allowed for your emotional reactions, you are still likely to have to make important decisions about treatment before you have had time to recover fully from the shock. You may be immediately offered major surgery, radio-therapy or chemotherapy – about which you probably know little or nothing. However, you need to go home, regain composure and think about things before making decisions about possible treatment. In particular, find out the *aims* of any proposed treatment. However, most doctors recognize that at this point you need thinking time; time to talk to relatives and friends; to consult with your GP and attempt to understand the aims and implications of the proposed treatment before making a decision. What you need to know is whether the treatment suggested is likely to lead to cure, or whether it is aimed at prolonging life or relieving pain and other symptoms.

Cancer and its treatment is a complex issue, and it needs to be realized that your doctor may not always be able to give you definite answers. What is important, though, is that there is time available for you to ask your questions and discuss the responses.

### Some suggestions for questions to ask your doctor/consultant

- Is the tumour/condition benign or malignant?
- If it is cancer, what kind do I have?
- If cancer, has it spread?
- What treatment do you propose?
- Can you predict how successful the treatment will be?
- What are the possible side-effects of the treatment?
- Can I have a second opinion? (Remember, a diagnosis and a proposal for treatment are not necessarily absolute. They are opinions, and another doctor may take quite a different view of the same symptoms and the method of treatment. If major surgery is suggested, then it is wise to ask for a second opinion.

One surgeon may be able to achieve the same results with less invasive surgery than another. Your consultant may even encourage a second opinion if he feels that it will reassure you. If he is not happy with your request, then by all means take up the matter with your GP. Do not be put off.)

- [If surgery] Will I need further treatment?
- Will it be possible to resume normal activities after the surgery?
- [If chemotherapy] What side-effects will there be?
- Can I get help with these side-effects?
- How often will I need further check-ups?
- What should I tell friends and relatives?
- What should I tell my employer?

Asking questions is an important part of the medical process, and ensures that you continue to recognize your own worth as a human being. *You are a person*, not a body to be handed over for others to do with what they will – no matter how good their intentions!

## Goals of treatment

Treatment is very complex, depending on the particular type of cancer, the stage of its development, and the general health of the individual. Whatever treatment is used, it is more effective when given as early as possible when the tumour is small and there is no detectable spread. However, this is not to say that treatment is ineffective even in the more advanced, secondary (metastatic) cancers. Many cancers can be cured outright; in other cases, it is possible to bring about long-term remissions or reduce the likelihood of recurrence or spread, and thus render the cancer more likely to be cured.

Treatments may also be used to slow down the rate of growth or to alleviate symptoms such as pain.

## The concept of cure

Some cancers, such as non-melanoma skin cancers and *in situ* cervical cancer, are highly curable. However, the word 'cure' has to be used cautiously in the case of other cancers, for the nature of the disease makes it difficult to pronounce a cure with certainty. This is because the progress of cancer is unpredictable. Following an apparently successful course of treatment there may be further growth, which may proceed slowly or at an accelerated rate. Because of this uncertainty it is common to refer to 'survival rate', meaning those people who can expect to survive five years or more. This five-year survival is often equated with a 'cure', and some patients consider that once they have passed the five-year mark they are 'home and dry'. However, with many, the anxiety remains that the disease will recur sooner or later. In fact, after five years without symptoms the chances of recurrence are markedly diminished, so far as many types of cancer are concerned. Two years is sufficient time to pronounce a cure in the case of Burkitt's Lymphona and testicular cancer, but eight to ten years is a more realistic estimate for such cancers as melanoma, breast, thyroid, or bladder cancer. Even with these more persistent cancers, the chance of recurrence decreases with each year.

It must be stressed that five-year survival is not an arbitrary figure. It is arrived at as a result of follow-up studies of many patients who have undergone treatment, and is a useful guide to measuring the successful outcome of treatment. Remember, cancer is unpredictable, and just as treatment is tailored to each individual, the specific cancer, its size, and rate of growth, the outcome must also be assessed on individual reactions.

It can never be said with certainty that after five years someone is cured. A single cell may escape treatment only to reproduce and spawn cancer some ten to fifteen years on. Most treatments (particularly chemotherapy) are, after 20 years, still being assessed and refined. Because there is difficulty in being dogmatic about the outcome of treatment, it is easier for the medical profession to talk in terms of 'no evidence of disease' and 'remission'. Full remission means that there is no evidence of cancer according to current investigation techniques. The medical profession is rightly cautious to use these terms for some time after treatment is finished. In spite of this caution, there is growing evidence that even in cancers that only a few years ago had poor prognoses, it is becoming increasingly more possible to talk in terms of longer survival rates and – possibly – a cure. Even though treatment may produce side-effects that are severe, most people feel this is worthwhile, particularly if after some months they can enjoy an acceptable quality of life for some considerable time.

## Palliative treatment

Where complete removal of a cancer, or a cure, is not a realistic goal, treatment may be given which aims at controlling the cancer or maintaining a good quality of life for as long as possible. This is known as palliative treatment.

The practice of palliative care therefore aims at:

- relieving undue suffering;
- enhancing the quality of life;
- encouraging the patient to abandon passivity and actively participate in the treatment process.

Even when it may not be possible to cure or produce full remission, cancer may be controlled. Treatment may be focused on stopping or slowing down the growth of a tumour or shrinking it, in order to alleviate pain or bleeding or to remove an obstruction. The result of such treatment is that many people feel better; and as a result are able to develop a more positive outlook on life, free from the exhausting effects of pain and unpleasant symptoms.

Because of increasing survival rates and the fact that many people still have the illness, albeit controlled, for some years (ten years or more in some cases), cancer could now perhaps be referred to as a chronic illness – not curable, but treatable, and not immediately life-threatening. During this chronic stage it is possible for many people to maintain a normal pattern of life. Until recently the chronic illnesses have usually consisted of heart problems, arthritis, emphysema, and multiple sclerosis. Such illnesses cannot be cured, but they can be controlled. With care, possible lifestyle changes, and appropriate treatments, people with these illnesses can function well. Today, as a result of palliative care, many cancer sufferers now come into the same category. In fact, it has become such an important part of cancer treatment that it is recognized as a specialism in its own right.

Palliative treatment may involve surgery, radiotherapy, nerve blocks to deal with pain, chemotherapy or hormone therapy, deep relaxation, exercise, or social activity – in fact, anything that is likely to improve the patient's lifestyle. Any decision about palliative treatment takes into account the severity of the symptoms, age, and general health, and weighs these against the adverse effects of the treatment.

Ideally, all aspects of therapy should be discussed with one or

21

more people who are close to you the patient, and who will be involved during treatment. They are the ones on whose support you will rely at all stages. At various times it may be necessary for a whole network of helpers to be involved in supporting you during and after treatment.

# 3

# Investigations and Different Types of Treatment

## *Forms of investigation*

The doctor's initial examination and questioning about your symptoms will help him decide whether further investigations are necessary for some disease process that may or may not include cancer. Symptoms that may appear unimportant to you may give the doctor clues as to the way in which he needs to progress. The doctor's physical examination is able to determine whether or not there are lumps or masses, and the form these take in various parts of the body. Your doctor may carry out a blood test himself, or he may refer you to the local hospital pathology department. This is only one part of the diagnosis, and it may be that results from several blood tests will be necessary.

X-rays and scans may also be used as an aid in making a diagnosis. Modern methods offer much more precision in locating the site of anything that is going wrong. Ultra-sound examinations allow precise measurements to be taken. Other examinations allow the consultant to look directly inside the body by means of a fibre-optiscope, e.g. gastroscopy, which allows a tube to be inserted via the mouth directly into the stomach. At the same time, the doctor may take a sample of tissue for examination; this procedure is known as a biopsy. The tissue removed can then be examined under the microscope and will give an indication as to whether or not there is evidence of cancer in that tissue.

## *Types of treatment*

There are a number of treatment options. These include:

- surgery
- radiotherapy
- chemotherapy
- hormone therapy
- combination treatments

There is no single form of treatment that applies to all cancers or all patients. The skill of the cancer specialist is to select at the outset the most appropriate form of treatment for you. Because there are so many different kinds of cancer affecting different parts of the body, the particular treatment you receive is determined by the characteristics of the particular type of cancer that has been diagnosed. Treatment decisions will be influenced by whether or not the tumour is large or small, and whether it is localized or has spread to other areas of the body.

### Surgery

Surgery is the primary and most effective treatment for most of the major types of cancer, and in the case of localized solid tumour cancers, it may be the only treatment necessary to produce an effective cure. The object of surgery in these cases is to remove completely all traces of the malignancy; however, where there is reason to believe that the cancer has spread to other parts of the body, the object is to remove as much of the tumour as possible by surgery, and then follow up with radiation or chemotherapy to destroy the remaining cells.

There is always the possibility of spread even in cases of cancer that are detected early. Even so, a decision *not* to use radiation or chemotherapy may be made where it is considered that an otherwise healthy person has an immune system strong enough to cope with the remaining rogue cells. Surgery may also be used to remove metastases (those cancers that have already spread to other parts of the body), and for the easing of symptoms such as pain.

It is important that you find out from your doctor exactly what the surgery is for, how extensive it will be, and what effects surgery is likely to have on your quality of life afterwards. You will be asked to sign a consent form agreeing to the operation, and before doing so you should be completely satisfied that you understand the purpose of the surgery. Beware of any consent form that gives 'blanket cover' for exploratory surgery. It may be helpful when thinking about surgery to enlist the aid of one of the cancer advice agencies who have experienced staff on hand to explain fully what is involved in various kinds of cancer treatment. It is very rare that treatment is required so urgently that there is no time for such discussions to take place. You will find a list of the main cancer advice agencies at the back of this book. In some hospitals, nurse advocates are available to help communication between consultants and patients.

## Radiotherapy

Radiotherapy is localized treatment, and involves the use of a small quantity of radiation to bombard the cancer cells with rays or charged particles. Such radiation damages the ability of the cancer cells to reproduce, so in effect the tumour becomes sterile. One way of administering radiotherapy is from outside the body, via machines that are capable of producing radiation that penetrates deep inside the body without the use of probes or needles, and that can be so finely focused that the rays avoid healthy tissue as much as possible. Like surgery, this treatment is most effective when it can be used locally, but it does have the advantage of destroying the tumour without the disadvantages brought about by surgery. No organs are removed and no damage is caused to healthy tissue, which inevitably happens in surgery. Radiotherapy usually involves daily attendence at the hospital for a period of one to six weeks in order to complete the course of treatment. The number of visits will depend on the dosage you require. It is considered best to give frequent small doses of radiation spread out over a period of time rather than give large doses over a shorter period. Frequent small doses ensure that the cancerous tissues receive the maximum dose of radiation, while the overlying skin and normal healthy tissue is relatively unaffected. Each session will last only a few minutes and is painless.

Another form of radiotherapy is to implant radioactive isotopes, encapsulated in special tubes or needles, either directly into the cancer, or nearby. These isotopes can also be injected into an organ or into the bloodstream, where they go directly to the tumour. It does not work on widely spread metastases unless wide-field radiation is used, but this technique can have serious side-effects on healthy tissue. Cancers vary greatly in their sensitivity to radiation, and while it is highly effective for certain types of cancer, others do not respond so well.

As well as inhibiting the reproduction of cancer cells, radiotherapy can actually cause shrinkage of the cancer tissue. It is often the spread of the cancer tissue that can cause pain. Radiation therefore may be given to shrink the cancer in order to give pain relief or to remove an obstruction of an internal organ.

Although radiotheraphy is normally given on an out-patient basis, the distance you have to travel for appointments may mean that it is more convenient for you to stay in the hospital. Sometimes admission may be advised so that the treatment may be monitored more closely, although such an admission does not necessarily mean that your condition has deteriorated.

## *Chemotherapy*

Quite simply, chemotherapy means the treatment of disease with chemicals or drugs, although nowadays the term is used more to describe the treatment of cancer with drugs specifically developed in order to destroy malignant cells and tumours. Chemotherapy acts on all the body's cells, and the drugs used are transported around the body via the bloodstream. You may hear chemotherapy referred to as 'cytotoxic', because the drugs are toxic, or poisonous, to all cells, malignant or not. Because reproduction of cancer cells is rapid, a cytotoxic treatment is most effective. Single drugs may be used or a number may be combined in a cocktail. Chemotherapy is unique among the conventional treatments for cancer because only chemicals have the ability to circulate through the body and reach cancer cells that have broken away from solid tumours and spread to distant sites. These cells may be undetectable, and therefore inaccessible to local treatments. Chemicals are used in the treatment of disseminated tumours of the blood and lymph.

Chemotherapy is the only scientifically proven method we have that can reach every part of the body that surgery and radiation cannot reach, and even sensitive instruments cannot see.

Chemotherapy is usually given in small doses over a period of months. Treatment is given in this way in order to keep pace with and outstrip the reproduction of cancer cells, and at the same time to avoid overwhelming healthy cells with toxicity. The calculations needed are very precise and the combination of drugs and dosages for particular cancers have been developed over a long period. The doctor specializing in this form of treatment is known as an oncologist.

The drugs circulate throughout the body in the same way that the cancer cells do, by flowing through the bloodstream. Once the drug meets up with the cancer cell it attacks and destroys it. Almost all the drugs used in chemotherapy suppress cancer by somehow altering cells' DNA, and thus their ability to reproduce. Since DNA is most vulnerable to drug interference during the reproductive phases on the life cycle, cancer cells are more likely to be affected than the bulk of the body's normal cells, which reproduce at a much slower rate, thus the very characteristic that makes cancer so dangerous contributes to its undoing. Some drugs, therefore, have been developed that are lethal to cells only during a specific reproductive phase. Other drugs are able to sabotage the cells no matter what phase they are in. The aim is to ensure that as many cancer cells as possible are killed without sacrificing too many normal cells. If there is too little of the drug, then too few cancer cells are killed; if there is too much of it, then too many normal cells are destroyed.

Everyone comes to chemotherapy with a different set of physical characteristics, and everyone reacts in a unique way. The doctor will make changes in your treatment if the side-effects are too debilitating or if the drugs do not appear to be working well. Treatments are carefully paced, allowing enough time between treatments so that normal cells can reproduce and replace lost cells sufficiently quickly to maintain your body at an acceptable level of functioning. However, there must not be too much time between treatments otherwise the cancer cells can greatly recoup their losses.

Because normal cells can also be attacked by cytotoxic drugs, there are many potential side-effects. The most common of these are loss of energy, loss of hair, nausea and vomiting, and susceptibility to infection. Although at one time chemotherapy tended to be used only as a last resort, it is now being given early in the course of the illness because that is when it works most effectively. It may even be the first choice of treatment to actually cure certain cancers. Often, however, it is used in conjunction with surgery and/or radiotherapy. It may be used after surgery to attack those cancer cells that have escaped into the bloodstream and may be lurking away undetected in other parts of the body. It may also be used before surgery to reduce the size of a tumour. Even when chemotherapy does not achieve an outright cure, it may enable people to control their cancer for many years.

Attempts are now being made to 'tailor' drugs for particular patients. A sample of the cancer is taken and the cells are cultured in test-tubes. Several anti-cancer drugs are applied to the different groups of cells before treatment begins, to find out which are likely to be most effective. As this technique develops, a lot of the guesswork will be removed from treatment, thus saving time and limiting the side-effects for the patient.

New drugs are constantly being introduced, and more and more is becoming known about the effects of these drugs, the diseases they treat, and how to control the side-effects. A substantial body of knowledge has been established about how much to give, in what combinations, and for how long.

### Hormone therapy

This may accompany the other forms of therapy or be continued as a means of preventing a recurrence of cancer long after other treatment has finished. Normally, the hormone tamoxifen is given to women who have had treatment for breast cancer.

### Combination treatments

As the name suggests, your treatment may involve surgery, chemotherapy, radiotherapy, and hormone therapy, at different stages during your illness.

### Blood counts in chemotherapy

Blood counts provide important information about the progress of the disease and the effects of treatment. They are helpful in deciding how to pace your treatment, particularly when chemotherapy and radiotherapy are being used.

Blood cells manufactured in the bone marrow are just as vulnerable to chemotherapy as the cancer cells themselves and many of the other cells of the body. Some of the drugs used in chemotherapy actually depress the activity of the bone marrow and influence its ability to reproduce blood cells rapidly enough to maintain good general health. Three different kinds of cells are produced in the bone marrow: red blood cells that carry oxygen; platelets that help blood clot and control bleeding; and white blood cells, which are part of the immune system and help fight off infection. During treatment, the blood count is closely monitored. A small sample of blood is usually taken so that it can be examined under a microscope to determine its quality. If the red blood cell count is low, then the person feels tired, weak, and listless. If the platelets have been reduced substantially, this means the blood cannot clot properly. When the white cell count is reduced, then the immune system is weakened. This means that the body is unable to fight off infection, and consequently the fight against the cancer cells is limited. Experience shows that blood counts reach their lowest level about seven to ten days after a treatment, and if no complications set in at this stage then the levels will be restored over the next few days. The blood count is very important, as it is used as a guide in ascertaining whether or not there should be any changes in the types and dosages of drugs used. If the blood counts become too low, then treatment may be temporarily reduced or withheld.

What is important for you, the patient, and your family during treatment is that you note any periods of tiredness and weakness. These are times when there is a need to reduce activity, to get more rest, and to limit involvement in anything that can cause stress. This is the time to listen to your body and go with the feelings.

Infections during cancer treatment pose the greatest threat, and it is important to report even the mildest of infections to your doctor. This is not a time to worry about 'bothering the doctor'. An infection treated at an early stage may be nipped in the bud; if not, it may have serious consequences, and your chemotherapy may need to be suspended while you recover from the infection. It is important to look out for high temperature, feeling chilled or shivery, loose bowels for longer than two days, burning during urination, coughing, sore throat, chest pains, shortness of breath, or any unusual discharge or blood from the urinary tract, the lungs, rectum, or vagina. Infections are usually treated with antibiotics, and the aim is to keep patients out of hospital. Sometimes antibiotics are administered as a safeguard against infection if there is a suspicion that a patient is particularly susceptible because of the type of cancer or their reaction to the treatment. Because of the risk of infection, patients are usually given a lot of precautionary advice about specific ways of avoiding problems.

# 4

# A Family's Story

In dealing with the day-to-day medical aspects of cancer, it is easy to underestimate the emotional impact on various members of the family and the need for support. Asking for outside help certainly does not mean we are inadequate or weak. On the contrary, if you can enlist help at a time of crisis, you can conserve your own much-needed energy. Generally speaking, people who cope well with their lives usually cope well at all stages of cancer. However, just because someone is resourceful and flexible and has a lot of inner strength does not mean that they are immune to the damaging effects of stress. Everybody needs help at some time or other; and it is those people who give the outward appearance of coping who may in fact be the most vulnerable, because they are unwilling or unable to admit to their own confusion and inner turmoil.

During one interview I asked Diane, who was in lengthy remission, how she had coped. Her answer was, 'Everyone expected me to cope – so I just had to get on with it!' In fact, she did cope extremely well, and subsequently recovered to continue bringing up her family. Throughout her illness, Diane kept all her fears and anxieties to herself. However, although she is now physically well, bottling up her feelings has taken its toll, and she has needed lengthy treatment for depression. Diane sees her depression as a weakness in her own character, and is having difficulty appreciating that it is probably the result of her own stoic attitudes in keeping things to herself in order to protect others.

The following stories have been included to illustrate how the impact of cancer influences people in a number of family situations. Everyone is affected differently, and you will see from the stories that people are affected according to the role that each one has to play, their age, stage of development, and status within the family. The differences also relate to the impact on the individual's personality and the natural resilience of that person. This will become clear as you read on . . .

## *Peggy's story* . . .

'Eight years ago, when our Maureen was 14, she was operated on

all of us. I know I should be thankful that Maureen survived – and I am really. My doctor keeps an eye on me and when I get too low, he gives me some tablets that pick me up. What seems to help me most is the local cancer fund-raising group. We are nearly all parents of children who have had the illness in one way or another. I can talk to them because they know what it is like.'

Peggy went on to talk about the rest of the family, and her feeling that somehow everything had changed with Maureen's illness.

'Arthur is a carpenter, and he was very excited about starting up on his own. He did this for about a year before Maureen was ill – of course, when she was in hospital he had to let a lot of his regular work go. He did not want the other two kids to be on their own for too long after school, but he is an independent man and didn't want to be a burden on the neighbours. I suppose but for him they'd have run wild, and the house would have been in a mess with me away from it.

'About six months after Maureen came home I could see Arthur was very low. He was very quiet and he didn't have very much get-up-and-go – didn't go after the work like he used to. Then he had trouble with the taxman – his books had got into such a mess. His business was very shaky, and we were finding it hard to manage with the payments on the house and the van. It got so bad that he was having to pay cash for all the work materials. He was never a man for drink either – just a pint with the lads on a Friday, and always home by 10 o'clock. He then started going out in the week – always said he was seeing somebody about a job, but I know he was drinking because I could smell it on him when he came in. He soon stopped that when the police picked him up for drink-driving – he lost his licence for six months. That pulled him up sharp!

'But for his mates helping him move stuff round from job to job, his business would have gone bust. It meant he could only do local odd-jobbing. He was at his lowest then, but he never said what was bothering him. Then, one night when we were in bed, he started to cry. I'd never seen him cry before, but he did, and I just held him close and I cried too. It seemed to go on all night, and though he still never said anything – he's not really a man for putting things into words – it must have got things off his chest. He must have had a lot building up inside him that we didn't know of. He has been better since, but I can see changes in him. Sometimes he is like a man just going through the motions of living. He gets mad at times, and when he does, it seems to be Gareth who catches it. Sometimes Gareth asks for it, mind you, because he can be cheeky to me and his dad. All Gareth wants to do is hang around with his mates, and he treats the house like a hotel – coming and going as he likes and never lending a hand with the housework. He can't hold down a steady job.

'Arthur seems to put most of his energies into his business by working long hours, and it upsets him to see Gareth wasting his time. Now that I think about it, Jenny and Gareth must have had a terrible shock themselves when Maureen was so ill, and I just took off and left them for so long. After all, I had always been there for all three of them – they never had to do anything for themselves. Everything was so ordered in our house. During the whole time Maureen was ill I must admit that I never really worried about them too much, as I was totally wrapped up in Maureen and the feeling that I was going to lose her. The only things I remember worrying about was that they should have clean clothes ready for school on Monday morning. It was only later, when Maureen had been home for some time, that I began to realize just what an effect the whole business had had on them. Teachers told me just how badly their school work had been affected, and from that time on neither of them seemed to do as well at school as I had been led to believe they might. I know that Jenny could easily have done well enough to be a teacher, but she refused to stay on at school and went to work with a local hairdresser. She got engaged on her eighteenth birthday and is hoping to be married in the next six months.'

## *Arthur's story . . .*

'When Maureen was taken ill I felt completely numb, cold inside. I am not much of a talker, but I think I talked even less during the whole time she was in hospital. It was as if I was holding my breath . . . waiting . . . Those three months seem blurred now. Peggy stayed with Maureen – she would have it no other way – and I acted as a sort of backstop at home. I could have done with Peggy back here sometimes, though, because the other two were very upset. Jenny cried herself to sleep every night – wanted her mam. Sometimes Gareth disappeared on the way home from school, and the neighbours would meet me from work with the news that he hadn't turned up for his tea. In spite of being tired, hungry, and worried, I would have to go out looking for him – most times I would find him in an old shed on the allotment. He said he just wanted to be on his own. His mam had never left either of them before, and I was at my wits' end what to do to console them. I kept this from Peggy because I didn't want to upset her any more than necessary. She had enough to do as it was.

'It is at a time like this when you really feel the need of the family around you, but of course Peggy is an only child and both her parents are dead. I've got a younger brother and his wife – they've got no children. They only live 20 miles away, but both of them work and they didn't offer to help with the children. They came on the phone every week full of excuses about how busy they were. It was either Bob's golf, Jean's amateur operatics, or stomach upsets – I stopped listening to the excuses after a bit. It was obvious that they couldn't handle the thought of Maureen's illness – but it did make me upset, because up till then I always felt we were close, that I could depend on them.

'The amazing thing is that after Maureen came home they kept making the point that if I'd only let them know how difficult things were, they could have helped out with shopping and transporting me to hospital, or taking the children out for the weekend. It just didn't make sense to me – they knew all along what the problems were, yet they still kept their distance. I've not had any time for them since. It still hurts that I had to rely on neighbours, and not family, at a time like that.

'Work was a struggle – my heart wasn't in it. I have never been very good at paperwork, and that was the first thing to go. It just piled up and piled up – sometimes I'd get it out on the kitchen table to sort through it, and then just push it to one side. I hadn't the heart even to look at it, and it all seemed so unimportant – and besides, every night there were the phone calls. A call from Peggy to give me the news from the hospital – and most of the time there was not much change. Still, it was enough to know that Maureen was no worse. Then there were the other calls from friends, neighbours, and my elderly aunts who wanted to know every detail – they seemed endless. I repeated over and over again what Peggy had told me – very rarely did I have time to finish my evening meal. I often ended up by eating the cold remains of it before I went to bed. I didn't sleep much – I was tossing and turning, up and down to the kitchen making cups of tea. At the end of three months of this routine and doing the hospital run every weekend, all normal living had disappeared. There seemed to be little point in it all. It was great when we heard that Maureen was on the mend and coming home. Now Peggy could come home too, and perhaps things would get back to normal.

'My worries about Maureen then became worries about how we would manage. My business was in a bad way, much worse than Peggy ever realized. I had borrowed money against the house to see us through, because I was only able to do about half the work I had been doing before, and I found the cost of housekeeping much higher than I expected. The taxman was soon on my back.

'I thought that when Maureen was home I would be able to catch up by doing extra work and soon be able to pay back the loan, but when that time came I was so tired that I felt as if over the three months I had changed from being a young energetic man, full of ambition for the future, to a tired old man with no energy left – jobs that once took me an hour to finish now took three hours. I felt so depressed, and what made things worse was that I had thought things would quickly get back to normal once Maureen was out of hospital. Instead, I found myself weepy, especially driving in the van between jobs. Sometimes I'd just drive up the hill and sit staring out at nothing in particular. There was a time when instead of visiting people to do estimates in the evening, I'd just call in the pub and sit drinking until closing time – it was only when I lost my driving licence that I realized how bad things had got. I seemed to have lost all contact with everybody. I don't think Peggy noticed it too much for a time, because she was still so involved with Maureen and sorting the house out, and doing her charity work. There were times when Peggy and I hardly saw each other – just as it had been when Maureen was in hospital. Of course, our physical relationship disappeared altogether when Maureen was in hosiptal, and it's never really got going again. We are both always so tired and we've got too much on our minds.

'I could never talk about my worries to anybody – people have enough worries of their own to listen to mine. I don't know what I'd have done without my mates when I couldn't drive the van, because Peggy doesn't drive. I would have felt so ashamed if we had had to give up the house and the business, and if the family had suffered because of me – after all they'd been through. I feel as if I just have to carry on working to make things up to them. When things get on top of me, I go for a good long walk on the hills.

'I keep telling Gareth how important it is that he should pull his weight in the house, but his attitude is "live for the day". I wouldn't mind, but he is a lad who could have gone places. Still, Maureen has come through well enough. She is a girl with spirit, and she's a fighter. In a way, it's Jenny I feel sorry for – she has had to fend for herself a lot more. She has learned to make her own way, though, and has a good job as a hairdresser. She has just got engaged to a nice lad, and they are hoping to save up enough money to get married this year.

'I still worry about Maureen, but it's no good talking about it all the time – you just have to get on with life. I don't think Peggy will ever get over Maureen's illness – she keeps re-living it over and over again. Jenny hopes to get married at Christmas, and that is just a few weeks before our Silver Wedding anniversary. I am thinking of surprising Peggy by booking up a winter holiday somewhere warm. Business is good now, and it's about time we had something fresh to look forward to. Maureen is well able to fend for herself for a week or two, and it will do her good not to have her mother fussing around.'

## *Gareth's story . . .*

'I was twelve when Maureen was taken ill, and I suppose the period when she was in hospital was when it dawned on me that I was no longer a child. It was the first time that I really realized bad things could happen to people, and although it was Maureen who was in hospital, it was my first experience of something very nasty happening to me. My world got turned upside down, and things have never been the same since. Everything I had relied on up 'til then just disappeared – Mam wasn't at home for what seemed ages, and our friends' mothers took turns to give Jenny and I our tea.

'Nobody would talk about Maureen and what was wrong with her – just that she had to go away to hospital because she was ill and needed an operation. I can remember Jenny and I talking about whether we would catch what she'd got, but no one would say what it was she had. My friend's mum was all right, but the house was smelly and they never had a tablecloth on the table. I never really fancied meals there – I remember going to hide in the old shed on the allotment with a bag of crisps.

'Maureen seemed funny when she came home. She was only two years older than me, but she seemed much older – she was so frail and white, and she had no hair. I had never seen a bald child. In other ways, she seemed so much more mature, and knew a lot about things I had never heard of. I know she got upset very easily at first, and I got told off if I made too much noise or jostled her. Mam expected me to take her to school when she started back, and she got really mad at me if I didn't bring her home again. If she saw us on the way home and I wasn't holding Maureen's hand, she would fly off the handle. And yet, because of this, the other kids would laugh at us – and this would make Maureen cry. I can remember at this time I used to get into quite a bit of trouble at school for daydreaming and not handing in my homework. In fact, Mam had to go to school about it. Dad and I used to get on well, but since I've grown older we don't seem to hit it off.

'After what happened to Maureen, I don't think you should plan too far ahead – just enjoy yourself while you can. You never know what's round the corner. I can always get work if I want it. I enjoy helping out on the farms in the summer. Just lately I have been doing a bit of bar work at night – it gets me out of the house. It's time I made my own way in the world, and I think I might try the army or the police. I don't want to stay at home for ever. We don't seem to be right as a family since Maureen was ill – somehow, we have separated.'

## Jenny's story . . .

'I was only ten when Maureen was taken ill. I don't really remember many of the details of that time, but I do remember crying myself to sleep because I thought I'd lost my mam and felt very frightened at what was happening. I knew Maureen might die, and dying seemed such a terrible thing. No one ever told me what was happening at the hospital, and I imagined all sorts of things. Somehow, during the time when Mam was away so much, I think I must have learned to manage on my own. Dad got us up in the morning, then we dressed and got our own breakfast before we got off to school. Dad seemed sad most of the time – his smile had gone, and I have never really seen it come back. I think it was round about then that we stopped having family outings like picnics or drives to the seaside, and we all seem to have gone our own ways since.

'Maureen seemed so much older than me when she came back from hospital. I don't know how she copes with Mam fussing around her all the time – until recently, she seemed to have no life of her own at all. I couldn't have stood it! I'm so glad that I met David – we get on really well together, and we have great plans for the future. I know Mam was disappointed that I didn't stay on at school, but I'm doing well at hairdressing and we hope to be able to set up a small business after we are married.'

## Maureen's story . . .

'I don't remember much about the time I was in hospital – I suppose I was too sick to be frightened or even to care. I certainly didn't feel I was going to die – it's only *since* then that I realize just how near I came to dying. The doctors have told me they are keeping an eye on things to see that it doesn't happen again – what bothers me is that it might. I get depressed when I think about the illness, so over the years I've learned not to dwell on it too much, and to make sure I keep my mind on other things. I know just how much Mam and Dad have done for me, but I just wish that Mam would let me do more for myself – she's so fussy about me.

'The worst part for me was in the first year or two after I came back home. My walking was awkward, my voice was peculiar, and I used to get very tired. My hair soon grew back, and I stopped being a nine-day wonder in the village, but I could never really get back on the same footing with my friends. Our interests seemed different, and they seemed so childish. I had spent a lot of time talking to adults, particularly the nurses. School didn't seem to interest me any more – it was for kids – and the teachers and the rules seemed so petty. I used to feel like screaming when they went on about uniforms, wearing hats, underlining headings . . . all these things seemed so unimportant after what I'd been through. Thank God, at least they let me get on with reading whenever I felt like it. I just kept out of their way, and sat my time out until I was 16. I suppose in a way you could say my schooling stopped at 14 – my only regret is that no one thought I was fit enough to take a job as soon as I left school. I'm sure I could have done something useful, even if only part-time. I became impatient with the people trying to help me. Sometimes I'd cry through sheer frustration that I wasn't able to make proper contact with my friends again. In fact, it was amazing that they still called round to see me. I suppose a lot of the frustration came from hearing them talk about their plans for the future, going to college, getting jobs, having boyfriends. All that seemed out of reach for me.

'I can remember spending long hours in my room feeling a

tremendous rage inside me, sometimes beating the pillow, sometimes even wishing I were dead. I spent a lot of time talking to Gareth – we get on well together. He seems to understand what I went through, and he treats me like a normal person. Jenny has always been independent, and we have never really been close. She never complains – just gets on with things in her own way, and everything seems to turn out right for her in the end. She knows what she wants and I admire her for it. I wish I was more like her.

'One of the worst things is that Mam has wrapped me up in cotton wool. Until a couple of years ago, she wouldn't even let me out on my own. I know that she's got this worry that I might get ill again – and the way she acts got me thinking for a long time that it was only a matter of time before I did. I was so frightened that I went along with her when she protected me, because I thought, somehow, that what she was doing might stop me from being ill again. However, I know a lot more about it now, and I know that living an ordinary life won't make any difference one way or the other. What will be, will be!

'Mam always insisted I go out with her to the shops – she would link arms in case I fell, and generally treated me like an invalid. We had loads of rows about this – and I would usually end up going off to my room to calm down. She called it sulking.

'Over the last two years, things have improved – the only sign there is anything wrong with me now is that I drag one of my legs a bit when I'm tired. I talked to the minister at church about how frustrated I felt, and how I thought I was ready to get out into the world – and maybe find a job and begin to have some independence. He has helped me a lot to see things more clearly. The illness may come back, but I am not going to have much of a life if I let worries about that get on top of me – as it seems to with Mam. Besides, everybody has to take some risks in life. I know that if I don't, I could go through the whole of my life, no matter how long it is, without really living – only existing. And it may never happen again anyway, and I would have given up all my chances.

'Since I have been going to the theatre group and started work, I find I am capable of a lot more than I thought I was. Mam doesn't know it yet, but I am thinking it is about time that I got a place of my own. She thinks my moods are connected to my illness, but they're not – I only get them when she tries to run my life. I seem to get on well with people outside of the family – it's nice to be with people who take me at face value and don't know my past history. I did think there was no way I'd ever have a boyfriend, what with my illness and being kept at home so much, but I have met some very nice men at the theatre group and find that I get along with them very well. I don't go out with anyone in particular, but we have dances and they make me feel completely normal. Recently, I have been able to put my foot down over the hospital visits. It was so embarrassing hearing Mam going on about my illness to anyone who would listen – not only the medical staff, but other people in the waiting-room. She would compare case-notes with other mothers, and start to offer them advice. Every time we visited the hospital, Mam would always find an opportunity to see the doctor on her own. I don't know what they talked about, but it frightened me no end thinking she might be told something about me that wasn't good, and that they were keeping it from me. It's a lot better now that I see the doctors myself – I'm in control. I know Mam doesn't want to break the links with staff at the hospital who were around at the time she was staying there – I think she likes to keep the contact going just in case . . . a sort of insurance policy.'

# 5

## Impact on Children
## and Young People

No one should underestimate the impact of the confirmation that there is a life-threatening illness in the family. It is overwhelming. As Arthur said, he was numb . . . cold inside. Peggy had thoughts only for Maureen and the fear that she was going to lose her. This dominated her so much that virtually everything else, even her two younger children, were put out of her mind. This is no reflection on her as a mother; this is a perfectly normal reaction. Peggy felt that no harm could come to Maureen while she stayed by her side, and she believed it was her place to be with her sick daughter. Neither Arthur nor Peggy was capable of making the sort of decision that an impartial observer might make. They both knew that something had to be done to maintain the household and the other children, but Arthur was not really capable of doing it, such was his state of shock, and yet, like an automaton, he struggled on – getting into more and more of a mess. He's not a man to shout out his troubles from the rooftops, and instead he internalized all his anxieties.

The younger children, Gareth and Jenny, felt abandoned, confused, and terrified. It had all happened so quickly. Gareth sought the security and comfort of his Dad's allotment shed, which offered him some privacy – where no one could see him if he cried.

Jenny's memory of the initial impact is blurred. This may be because time has had this effect, or may be because she has 'blanked out' the real impact of the shock. This often happens with children; it is a sort of protective measure that comes into play, and stops them experiencing the full impact. It can be very painful to have to cope with the realities of a bad situation, and blanking out stops you from being overwhelmed with fear and anxiety. Although Jenny cried herself to sleep, people around her believed she was taking things very well.

There is evidence that Jenny is a coping girl who gets on with things, and this is the reaction of many children who have experienced some kind of trauma in their lives. They do not betray what is truly happening inside them, and it may be that years later –

when they develop a depression, an anxiety, or some symptoms of illness – that the feelings bottled up in childhood will surface.

Recently, I was consulted by a young woman called Anna in her late twenties who was a compulsive eater of chocolate. This caused her great concern – for she spent two or three pounds buying chocolate on her way to work, and ate all this before the morning tea-break – when she again stocked up with more chocolate bars. These would be gone by lunchtime; she would then eat a full lunch and several more bars of chocolate. Anna ate her way through four or five more chocolate bars in the course of the afternoon, and would still be 'bingeing' while driving home. When her husband arrived home he would ask Anna if she had been a good girl, and had kept away from the chocolate. She always replied 'Yes' and was then rewarded by . . . a box of chocolates! Anna had got to the point of realizing that she needed help, because her chocolate-eating was out of control. She hated herself for deceiving her husband. The surprising thing was that she had not put on extra weight, and still had a clear, healthy complexion. During therapy, it transpired that at the age of three, her mother, a single parent, had died suddenly; and of course Anna had felt immediate abandonment. At that age she was not aware of what death meant – all she knew was that her mother had gone away. She was looked after by her mother's sister and husband, who brought her up as their own. To all intents and purposes, Anna had made a good recovery, and showed no signs of emotional upset. She did well in school and got a job as soon as she left, as an administrator in local government. During her therapy sessions, it was possible to get Anna to re-live the feelings relating to the loss of her mother, and she talked of feeling cold and empty inside. She recognized that these feelings had often recurred throughout her childhood and adult life, making her feel 'very odd'. It was this empty feeling that prompted her need for chocolate; and it seemed that chocolate was the only thing to remove it. Of course, as time went on, the feeling remained, no matter how much chocolate she ate, as she was not addressing her real problem.

It would appear from Jenny's and Gareth's stories that they never seemed to get back on to the same footing with their parents after Maureen's illness. Mistrust can remain long after the feeling of abandonment is over, even when the 'abandonment' has been unavoidable.

Some years ago, in my early days as a social worker dealing with children's problems, I was called in to see a family where the 12-year-old son had developed a pattern of school truancy. The interesting thing about his behaviour was that he rarely went further than the end of his own road, where he found himself a suitable hiding place to watch his own house. Finding this hiding place uncomfortable and cold on long winter days, he discovered a new one: he sneaked back into his house at a suitable opportunity, and hid himself under the table in the front room. The table was completely covered by a chenille cloth, which almost touched the floor. The room was rarely used, except at weekends, so he felt safe.

In exploring this situation with the family, it appeared that the truancy usually happened when his father was not at work, but was at home alone with the boy's mother. The parents had put this down to some jealousy of the relationship between his parents. However, further discussion brought out the fact that some five or six years before, the mother had gone into hospital with cervical cancer. The whole incident had been kept secret from the boy, and he had been given no preparation for his mother's admission to hospital. He experienced a sudden abandonment and, in his own mind, she had gone for ever; his security was completely taken away. The hospitalization involved his father taking time off work to organize his wife's admission, and make afternoon visits to the hospital.

Although not consciously aware of it, the boy's behaviour was quite rational. He associated Father being at home when he was at school as a signal that his mother was likely to disappear again, thus repeating the abandonment. All the boy could tell us was that whenever he had to go to school and his father remained at home, he felt frightened, knotted up inside, panic-stricken. However, simple explanation of the irrationality of his thinking would never relieve the boy's inner mistrust. The parents needed to begin a long process of regaining their son's confidence by becoming aware of their tendency to be secretive about many things that went on within the family. They needed to become much more open in their communication with him about all sorts of things, so that at all times he felt included. This tendency to wish to protect children from all that is bad may be an instinctive reaction on the part of the parents, fearing that their offspring may not have the capacity to cope with news of a parent's illness or impending death.

I suppose I felt some sympathy with this boy because my own memory tells me that at a similar age I was sent away to relatives – ostensibly, to enjoy the school summer holiday. It was a holiday that seemed to me to go on for ever, but I was not complaining. I was enjoying myself in the company of my aunt and uncle and cousins. Being an only child, I found the companionship of other children great fun. We went for picnics, and I remember seeing my first dragonfly when playing by a pond in the woods. The Sunday school, with the sun pouring in shafts of light and the congregation singing 'Tell me the stories of Jesus', still remains clear in my memory. One day, though, my idyll was shattered. My mother arrived without notice, dressed all in black, and looking very sad. She broke the news to me that my father was dead. This moment is probably the most vivid memory I have of my childhood; and looking back, this experience probably spelt the end of my childhood. It may well be that I had been told my father was very ill, or even dying, from cancer. I may even have seen him in bed, but I have absolutely no memory of this. The news of his death probably blanked out everything else. To me, it seemed that things were never the same again. I was different from other children. At this point, I lost even more than my father – I lost the intimacy of a child with its parents. I lost my trust in adults, and felt I was the only one who was not in on the secret. I felt disconnected.

Although I was welcome in the larger family group of grand-parents, aunts, uncles, and cousins, I still felt an 'outsider'. I realized, I suppose, that I had to protect myself from further hurt by not becoming too reliant on anybody. From that point on, I became less trusting and more independent, both physically and emotion-ally. Older members of my extended family will have their own memories of what it was like when my father was diagnosed, nursed, and died, but none will have experienced it in the same way as I did at the age of five.

In the case of Jenny and Gareth, what made it worse for them was the length of time involved during which their parents were totally preoccupied with other matters. They experienced, in their own personal way, a combination of what seemed to them emotional as well as physical abandonment; neither of them was helped by being 'farmed out' with different neighbours and school friends. Even though they felt sorry for their older sister, they also had feelings of intense sorrow for themselves. They may even have felt guilty about this. Or they may even have been angry with their sister for being ill and upsetting their family life. Then, of course, they might have felt guilty about that. There were comments that they never seemed to get back on the same footing with their parents after Maureen returned home. This can easily happen when children lose some of their trust in parents, and they feel it is safer to withdraw from such close dependence in case the whole thing happens again. They are protecting themselves for the future.

Although Peggy, their mother, was with them at weekends, her mind was elsewhere. Hence both Jenny and Gareth remained preoccupied with their loss; not able to talk about it, and receiving no help in expressing it. They were kept short of information, and fantasy filled the gaps.

Of course, as I am sure you will appreciate, as you read this, that Peggy and Arthur faced the sort of dilemma that every parent dreads facing, and their ability to think straight was extremely limited by the shock of the news of Maureen's illness. They had to judge between the needs of Maureen, and those of Jenny and Gareth. Ideally, it would have helped for Jenny and Gareth to have been looked after in their own home by a close relative or friend, who could offer consistency of care and security in their familiar territory. The compromise that was reached was satisfactory, but it did impose tremendous strains on the whole family.

There is a lot of evidence that young children who spend some time in hospital away from parents, or a consistent caring figure, suffer not only the illness, but the effects of separation and loss. They too feel the effects of abandonment, and in extreme cases it has been known for them to become so mistrustful of other people that they can become emotionally deprived to such an extent that they lose their ability to express or feel affection for others. It has become the practice in most hospitals to have a policy of open visiting for parents, and to encourage them to take over most of the day-to-day care of the child, while the hospital staff concentrate on the medical supervision of the child. This is very helpful in mitigating the depriving effects of hospitalization on the sick child, but of course, as we have seen, it places parents who have more than one child in a quandary. It would have been helpful in the case of Jenny and Gareth if they had been able to join both parents at weekends at the hospital, in order to spend some time with them and their sister as a family unit. Indeed, most hospitals now encourage this family involvement; and it is good to see that parents who have already been through similar experiences have taken the initiative and established hostel-type accommodation near some hospitals, so that families can get together and preserve essential links, particularly for those families living some distance away.

When children go into hospital, they need the comfort of a parent; and babies and young children may need this continually throughout their stay. In the case of older children, the reassuring presence is particularly important before, during, and after treatment sessions and surgery. At these times, anxiety is likely to be at its highest. In fact, older children, once the crisis is over, may well benefit from short periods without the constant attendance of the parent.

Although they had their problems, this family was fortunate in that it was a united family. Many children have parents who are not happy together, or who may have already separated, divorced, or even be remarried with new family ties. Children having the illness may be caught up in a struggle between warring parents, and it is not easy, in a situation where relationships are already strained to the limit, for estranged parents to reconcile their differences sufficiently to sort out what is best for the child – both from a practical point of view and from an emotional stance. In the best interests of all the children involved, it would seem that at an early stage one or both parents should seek the help and advice of the professional social work staff attached to the hospital.

Many children do have separated parents, but, as one parent said to me, 'When this happens to your child, everything else pales into insignificance.' The crisis of cancer at this time is likely to create a number of conflicts. It could be that the natural parent that no longer has custody may not even be told about the illness, or there may be real objections on the part of the parent having custody to the other parent rekindling an association with the child that was thought to have long since ended. New families are likely to have been created in the interim period, and if time and energy is switched from the second family to a child from an earlier relationship, there may be resentment or jealousy on the part of the new partner and their children. Even if no time is actually spent visiting the sick child in hospital, it could be that emotionally the separated parent diverts attention to the sick child. If one parent has not been a regular feature in the sick child's life for some time (whatever the reason behind it), it would not be in the best interests of the child for that parent suddenly to appear out of the blue. It is important to assess just how significant you are in the life of the sick child, and ask serious questions of yourself. For whose sake are you visiting? Yours or the child's? In the same way, the parent having custody also needs to be asking serious questions about what is in the best interests of the child. Is your own enmity towards your previous partner behind a decision to exclude *all* contact? These situations are a real test of maturity for separated parents – and particularly for the parent who has care and custody, because it is this parent who will be the final arbiter of the child's needs.

Children have a right to know about anything that affects the family – particularly something as serious as a life-threatening illness. They can sense when something is wrong, and if you attempt to protect them by saying nothing or making light of it, their fears may conjure up something worse. If you do not talk about the illness, it may suggest to the children that cancer is a subject so terrible that it cannot be discussed – and the end result may be that the children become overwhelmed by their fear. It is far better that they find out the truth from a loved one whom they trust than from a neighbour or school friend. If this happens, they may feel that someone in the famiy has completely betrayed their trust; they can feel isolated and left out. And those nursing the secret may increase their own isolation, and deny themselves a source of comfort.

It is important that we adults realize that children do have the capacity to deal with the truth – even when the truth is very sad. It is much better for children to know what they are up against than to live in a situation of uncertainty. When children are included and they know exactly why someone is upset – and that the illness is not their fault, but something that has to be faced – they can actually grow as a result of sharing the experience with other family members. Children are very sensitive to changes in the emotional climate in the home. They are resilient enough to cope with temporary changes: temporary changes in mood, short-term separations, times when adults seem preoccupied and have no time for them, physically or emotionally. These short-term negative experiences do not produce long-term problems for children; they have to learn to accept that they are not the centre of the universe, and that from time to time they have to fit in. What is important here is that the child understands the reasons for the interruption to the normal pattern of life.

However, it is a different matter if the illness is life-threatening and likely to involve serious surgery and treatment that may continue for a long time. When a parent, brother, or sister is hospitalized for a lengthy time, then the hospital should not be a place that exists in children's fantasies, but should be made a reality. They must see where the hospital is, see what room their loved one is in, and know something about the treatment and the likely effects of that treatment. This is particularly important if the treatment is going to change the physical appearance, or have short- or long-term effects on the way the patient is able to interact with them. Opportunities should be taken to spell out which changes are likely to be permanent, and which are likely to be short-lived and to disappear as healing takes place.

Children can often accept physical disability easier than adults. They don't need long explanations, but a short account of why someone looks or feels the way they do is important. The main thing is that children have a chance to see for themselves what is going on, and to have questions answered honestly and truthfully without too much elaboration and emotion. Children below the age of puberty can easily be overwhelmed with too much detail, particularly with some of the more gruesome aspects, so it is important to steer clear of these and to stick to straightforward and factual information. If you tell them too much, they become obsessed with the details.

What is difficult for everybody in the family when someone has cancer are the uncertainties, the unknowns. Once the immediate threat to life is over, then everybody will be living with uncertainty. It is part of the reality. There will be many questions that you will not be able to answer; and there will be many questions that your doctor will not be able to answer either. This just has to be accepted. How much a child wants to know will depend a lot on the particular child, and it is important – even with toddlers – that they should know that someone is ill and what treatment will involve.

It is important that children remaining at home when someone is hospitalized are cared for by a familiar person if possible. Young children fear separation and strangers, and being abandoned. There is no clear-cut age to define 'young children', but certainly the younger the child is, the stronger these fears – particularly if it is a parent who is taken into hospital. Older children, and even adults, can go through the same fears. The fear of separation, abandonment, and loss is basic to everyone, without exception.

Unwanted changes are challenges that upset the equilibrium, and everyone has a different capacity to cope with unwanted changes. When a challenge is new and there is no blueprint for coping with it, there will be a period of uncertainty – perhaps even panic, and attempts to solve problems with immature behaviour. Normal rational behaviour may be abandoned temporarily; when our equilibrium is upset, there will always be strong feelings.

Sometimes these feelings may be expressed as anger and rebellious-ness, sometimes the feelings may be internalized and show them-selves as disturbances in eating, sleeping, school work, and relationships. Gareth showed some evidence that he was coping with some internal emotional difficulty, and this was expressed in his daydreaming. Every teenager goes through such periods during their school life, but usually they are short-lived. The fact that it was sufficiently serious for the school to ask Peggy to call and talk to them about it indicates the depth of Gareth's problem. He is a sensitive lad, and at the time he was coming to terms both with Maureen's illness and his first intimation of mortality. He was also offering his sister protection and emotional support – a big task for a youngster just entering his teens. It is little wonder, then, that Gareth drifted off during school hours.

The teenage years are particularly difficult, as this is a time when young people can have strong emotional swings; and if there is a disturbance at this time, any balance they might have achieved can easily be upset. If teenagers are going through a period of rebelliousness against a particular parent while they are striving for independence, and this parent becomes ill, then this can be particularly upsetting for the young person concerned – who may even indulge in some magical thinking that the illness has got something to do with them. They may feel guilty that a parent is ill, especially if they have had bad thoughts about them. This is a time when they need to be reassured that the illness has nothing at all to do with them. The feelings may even be stronger if the parent has been wont to say in the past things like, 'You'll be the death of me', 'Everything would be all right in this house but for you', 'No wonder I'm a bag of nerves, the way you behave', or 'I'll be glad when you're off my hands'.

Restoring equilibrium will take time, and with time will come some adaptation to the new situation. It may not be the best adaptation, but it may be one that brings some degree of security. It often helps during these times of threat to keep on with routines that are familiar.

No matter who is ill in the family, it is important to try to keep things as normal as possible – that is, continuing with familiar activities, maintaining a regular daily routine like getting up at the same time, getting off to school, doing homework and, if possible, ensuring that if substitute care has to be provided, it is provided by the same person. The illness and its impact is bad enough without constant changes in personnel, homes, activities, and routines. This continuity of life is very important – not only for the children, but for adults too. There is no gain from throwing up everything in the face of the illness. Drastic change is OK for a short time, but it cannot be continued indefinitely; and, as we have already said, cancer is an illness that is indefinite in its outcome and in its duration.

Maureen's illness occurred at a crucial time in her life, a time when she would be moving away from childhood into adulthood. This is normally a time when young people are faced with many uncertainties about themselves and their future, particularly uncertainties about their physical appearance. The teenage years are those years when young people practise and gain experience in establishing relationships on an adult level. They gain confidence from successful encounters with people in the adult world, but at the same time they are fearful of appearing clumsy and tongue-tied or getting into a situation where they feel completely out of their depth. The culmination of this period is a move into employment, a move away from home, and a move into sexual relationships. Developmentally, Maureen's crisis coincided with facing the many challenges of growing up, and her illness interrupted this process. Even before her life really got going, she had to cope with the idea that it might be cut short at any time by a recurrence of her illness. At a time when her confidence was in the balance, her fears, anger, and frustration were increased as a result of the threat hanging over her. This is quite a burden to carry on the road to maturity. Because of her reduced capacities, which increased her isolation from her peers, Maureen felt different – indeed, *was* different, and she suffered a blow to her attempts to build up some self-esteem. She was denied the opportunity to pass the normal milestones of growing up.

When the future is uncertain, then it is difficult to make plans. At the very least, serious illness in adolescence is an interruption in normal development. Things have to be shelved and picked up later on after a period of healing and reassessment. Maureen's progress towards health was impeded by her fears and the fears of her mother, who was over-protective and over-controlling. By the age of 22, she was just beginning to achieve the goals normally reached at 16.

# 6

# Moving On

Returning home from hospital after surgery or intensive treatment for a life-threatening illness is a crisis in itself. It is a crisis that involves facing up to yet more change, and it imposes its own anxieties and fears. Returning home is the time when real grieving for the loss of a former life, physical capabilities, and mental capacities might start. Although returning home can be a cause for celebration, it can also signal a realization that members of the family, including the patient, are in a state of physical and mental exhaustion. It can also signal a period of real isolation.

When you have gone through serious physical illness, or have been caring intensively for someone suffering from it, you need a period of complete rest. In fact, the return home of the patient can often be the signal for the start of depression, although this depression is not necessarily to be equated with a clinical depressive illness. It is a depression of the body, the mind, and the spirit – in other words, everybody feels low, and everyone in the family needs a period of recovery, in which all are able to regain strength and energy and take stock of what has been lost from a former life. Put simply, each member of the family needs to consider how to begin to reshape the future.

Although this is the time when valuable psychological work needs to take place, the extra burden of looking after someone at home and adjusting to new roles, and the physical and emotional changes in the patient, means there is very little time or space to pause for breath.

## *Moving on can be difficult*

Maureen and her mother had spent three months tied into a hospital routine with supportive staff around them. In hospital, Maureen was one among a number of patients who shared similar experiences, but returning home meant that she and her mother and the rest of the family were left to cope alone.

Returning home is often the signal for a round of visits and attention, but the convalescent and family at this time can experience an inner feeling of isolation, a feeling of being cut off from other people as a result of their experiences. Maureen knew that her illness had left her looking and feeling different; her voice was different and she walked oddly. She felt other things had changed too. The relationship between herself, her brother, and sister was no longer the same; and she felt she had grown apart from her school friends, who now seemed to her very immature. When Maureen returned to school, her feelings of isolation were reinforced. She was behind with her work, and, with poor concentration and her energy level low, no one made any demands on her. To the other children, she was an oddity, and she had to face teasing. Clearly, she was a candidate for remedial teaching, which for some reason was not made available to her.

Maureen was growing up. She was an adolescent, a time when most children are beginning to move away from physical and psychological dependence on their parents. She also had her illness to deal with, and there was a lot of uncertainty as to its future direction. She needed time, space, and opportunity to gain confidence, and to recover some of her lost self-esteem. She had to reassess and accept her new physical image, and the fact that her experience had made her different from her school friends. Above all, she needed to be helped to make her way back into the real world by means of a series of small steps. She needed care, but not over-protection; challenges, but without being overwhelmed. Once she had got the energy to return to school, one of the most effective ways to help her take those small steps and to provide challenges would have been to set her work targets.

As a teenager, Maureen was in an odd relationship with her mother. Peggy had given so much to her and wanted to continue protecting her. She was obsessed by the fear that Maureen might be ill again, and these fears dominated the way she treated her. Therefore the dominant theme of Peggy's relationship to Maureen was *protection*. It is normal for an adolescent to express anger and rebelliousness towards parents as they move towards independence; Maureen was no different, but there was a big gap between what she could do and what she wanted to do at this crucial period of her life. It is no wonder that she withdrew for long periods, often suppressing the anger she felt towards her mother and her situation in general. It sprang not only from her frustration at her inability to achieve independence, but also from the feeling that her 'future' had been taken away from her.

Many people experience the unwelcome changes resulting from

life-threatening and disrupting illness. They find limitations on their ability to live as they would like to, and they experience anger and depression. When a person's future appears to have been taken away, the anger can become so strong that if it is not expressed appropriately, it can turn inwards and produce strong suicidal thoughts – and from time to time this happened to Maureen. These feelings of anger and depression are shared by many people with chronic, painful, debilitating illness. They feel angry when they compare themselves with the person they once were, and when they look into their future they can see nothing but a life that continues to provide uncertainty, pain, discomfort, and further limitations. They reach a stage when they can see no way forward. These feelings need to be recognized and acknowledged.

Maureen was helped by talking things over first with her brother, and then with her church minister, who helped her to see that she was a person in her own right. They helped her to put her illness and her life into some kind of perspective. Her period of emotional and spiritual healing took a long time, and this period can be prolonged if the need for emotional healing is ignored or accorded a low priority. Physical treatment of illness is only part of the process of restoring people to wholeness.

As she came through her crisis, Maureen was able to make some plans for the future. She continues to have 'moods' as her mother calls them, but she identifies them now, at the age of 22, not so much with her illness, but with the normal resentment of someone who resists other people interfering too closely in their lives. She has begun to see that in spite of what she has lost and in spite of the uncertainties relating to the possible recurrence of her illness in the future, she has to take some risks in order to live a full life. She knows it is time to move on.

Maureen's parents came through a very testing time during the critical three months of her illness. They came through relieved that their daughter survived the treatment, and, what is more, with comparatively little lasting damage. Maureen's homecoming was exciting, but their enjoyment was curtailed as they felt a sense of anticlimax. They were completely physically and mentally exhausted after their ordeal.

They faced a difficult period of readjustment. There were the ever-present worries about the future course of the illness. Other things bothered them too. They felt that the two younger children seemed to have grown away from them; and on top of all this, they had strong feelings about the fact that close family members had not rallied round as they might have expected. They were bitter, angry, and confused about this. Once the immediate crisis was over, Arthur had to repair his business and financial situation, which had deteriorated badly. It is no wonder that both parents, faced with so much, had a series of depressive episodes to deal with. It is normal for depression to follow a period of physical and emotional strain; it is nature's way of saying 'Ease up – it's time for a rest'. The problem is that when this happens, the depression brings its own devastation – especially if you know that there are things that must be done and yet you cannot find the energy to do them. Things pile up, and feelings of frustration, confusion, and helplessness can increase.

## Waiting for the 'other shoe to drop'?

Peggy is still waiting for a recurrence of Maureen's illness. She has spent years 'holding her breath' waiting to hear bad news. As a result, she is in a perpetual state of anxiety. Her solution seems to be to get some tablets from the doctor from time to time – perhaps what she really needs is the opportunity to sit down at regular intervals with someone who is willing to listen to all those things that are causing her anxiety and confusion. Peggy needs someone to 'mother' her, but she just has to soldier on. Not content with keeping the protective wall around Maureen and running the home, she then has to cope with her anxiety about the future by getting deeply involved in activities outside the home. Her busyness seems designed to keep her anxiety at bay. Once she stops, she feels, she might go to pieces. Her link with the hospital somehow indicates that she is keeping one hand on the lifeboat – just in case Maureen should ever need it again.

Emotionally, Peggy is completely absorbed in anxieties about Maureen's future. Everything Maureen does is judged in terms of whether or not it is 'safe'; thus her efforts have underlined Maureen's 'invalid' status. She has a very strong fear that Maureen could do something that might trigger off a recurrence – and nothing will reassure her that leading a normal life is the best thing. Maureen's normal adolescent behaviour and her struggle for independence has been overshadowed, and all her behaviour has been attributed to her illness. However, we are not condemning Peggy for this – her reaction is quite understandable.

Many parents will select one of their children for over-protection if they have had some illness or some slight defect as a child. Perhaps they have been asthmatic, needed glasses, or had a weak chest. The parents' over-protectiveness seems to serve to delay the move from childhood through adolescence to maturity. Even if she had not had her tumour, Maureen may still have been selected for the role of being protected.

Peggy could probably have been helped sooner by belonging to a support group where members listen to one another and support each other in various ways. As it is, she has involved herself with a group that keeps itself very busy planning fund-raising activities. It is almost as though this group has dedicated its members to repaying some debt that they feel they owe.

This over-emphasis of the mothering role has detracted from Peggy's role as wife. In the early stages, immediately following Maureen's return from hospital, it was only to be expected that both parents would be totally absorbed in their own exhaustion and worries, and have nothing left over for each other. Normally, the couple would resume their usual married relationship as they recovered their energy. Peggy, however, seems to have switched completely into the mothering role, with Maureen as the main target; and Arthur, the man who doesn't talk much about his feelings, is left in his own isolation.

## Feeling cut off

Clearly, Arthur is isolated. In the months following the illness he showed signs of breakdown, culminating in his unaccustomed drinking. He is not able to talk about his problems, and feels his situation all the more because he has this feeling that as 'the man of the house' he has to cope: to provide security and strength at all times for the rest of the family. It is a bitter blow to his pride when he sees that he cannot carry this burden alone.

Arthur was also harbouring strong feelings about being let down. Feelings of disappointment, anger, and confusion have forced him to review his relationship with his brother. It has been tested and found wanting. He thought he could depend on him for help at any time – after all, when his brother needed *him*, he was there to help!

Arthur's experience seems to be a common one. Most of us feel awkward, and wonder what to say and how to behave, when we come face to face with a friend or someone in the family who has been diagnosed as having a serious illness. Generally, we find the right words and the best way to offer whatever help and support is necessary. We know that unless we are very close to the patient, we don't have to bear the full burden; and that by taking on even a small task, we are offering considerable support.

However, some people are terrified of illness and just cannot cope with the feelings that it provokes in them. The feelings are so strong that they produce a state of panic, which causes them to flee from it – to distance themselves. They may telephone frequently rather than visit. It is probably an anxiety that needs some sympathy rather than condemnation. This exaggerated fear may be a legacy of some experience in their past; it is not only related to cancer, but to illness or hospitals in general. Sometimes it helps if the person with this fear can be asked to do some simple practical task that does not bring them into contact with the patient, sick room, or the hospital; but if this happens to be your problem, then you need to seek help with your phobia. Even discussing it with a good listener would be a useful starting point. It may be possible to cover up the fear in the short term, but in a long-term illness the fear may have the effect of causing the sufferer to sever relationships rather than face the actual fear. Illness occurs in every family, and it is a pity if family relationships are disturbed, sometimes for ever, if this fear is allowed to dominate. When the crisis of the illness is over and people with this fear feel they are no longer under threat, they may assume that they can pick up the threads of the relationship exactly the way it was before, and behave as if they have been fully involved in supporting the family and the patient. The problem is that when this happens in a close and otherwise caring family, it seems as though the person with the fear was completely unfeeling, uncaring, and selfish. All that it produces is a hurt that colours all future relationships with that family member; in Arthur's case it was his brother's problem that added to the burden of Arthur's depression.

## Easing depression

Arthur had to face his depression, and it is interesting that – in common with many other people – he copes with it in a non-verbal way. It helps him considerably to cling on to Peggy for physical comfort and to just let go. Many men bottle up their feelings and are reluctant to show them; boys are often trained in childhood to control their emotions – not to show fear and to hide their hurt. Fortunately, Arthur does allow himself, in the security and privacy of the marital bed, to release his feelings in tears. Physical closeness is very important to people who find difficulty expressing things in words. Being physically close to someone relaxes, brings reassurance, and takes away the feeling of isolation, and it is then possible to let things go – to release strong, pent-up feelings.

It is interesting also that Arthur, like many others, has found another way of easing his depression: he takes off to the hills and walks. You don't have to walk miles – probably about 2 miles' brisk walking is enough to enable a person to get a lot of oxygen into the system, and to release endorphins – the body's own natural morphine-like chemicals that counteract depression. Endorphins have the effect of making people feel good; but more than that, walking gives us the chance to experience at first hand the sights, smells, and sounds of the outdoors. The whole effect is a tonic –just looking at the sky as you walk usually produces a feeling of lightness, of well-being.

It seems that Arthur has now recognized that it is time for the family to move on; that there has been too much sadness and depression for too long, and that it has become a way of life for all of them. As Gareth indicated, they are a sad family. Arthur wants to break out of this, and Jenny's wedding seems an ideal opportunity for Peggy and Arthur to go on holiday and together enjoy a fresh start. He knows that the time has probably come for both of them to loosen the apron strings and start a new life for themselves.

Even though it seems as if many aspects of their lives have been shelved, in reality three children have moved out of childhood, through adolescence, and on to maturity. Peggy and Arthur have also been maturing and learning a new set of values; although before Peggy can move on properly, she needs some help in recognizing that Maureen doesn't need her 'mothering', and that her role needs to change. There are so many other things ahead of her to give her emotional satisfaction once Peggy learns to let go.

# 7

## Carers and Supporters

### *What is a carer?*

In recent times, the word 'caring' seems to have become synonymous with looking after in their own home someone who is ill, handicapped, disabled, or infirm through old age. It used to be called 'home nursing', and implies that something more is involved than ordinary nursing. The word 'caring' in this context suggests to me an essential emotional link between the 'carer' and the 'cared for'. Yet the 'carer' need not even be someone you know. There need not be any emotional link when you start, but this usually follows when people are so closely bound together.

The feelings involved may not always be positive, and the relationship may mean coming to terms with strong negative feelings that become established between the 'carer' and the 'cared for'. The process involves looking after the physical and emotional needs of someone who is going through a permanent or temporary period of dependence. Whatever they are called, a good nurse or carer always has an eye on encouraging recovery where this is possible, and working towards the maximum possible degree of independence and self-determination.

At all stages in cancer, family and friends are the major support system for a patient, and at various times may be called upon to respond to their needs in a multitude of ways. Every situation is different, and the illness may be such that the demands made on carers are comparatively light. However, this will very much depend on its severity and length. The kind of support needed will vary from being available to ease fears and anxieties, to providing practical help – such as shopping, or gardening, making sure household finances are secure, escorting to and from hospital visits, communicating the patient's requirements with professionals, full-time home nursing or daily hospital visiting, cooking, laundry, child-minding, doing the school run, companionship. You can probably add a lot more things to the list, depending on your own circumstances.

Although this book is concerned with helping everyone who is closely affected by cancer to cope with a number of associated crises and to suggest ways of managing the illness, this chapter is specifically addressed to 'the carer', regardless of whether this is a major live-in role or simply providing support to those who are in closest contact with the patient.

## Crisis points

Cancer, as we have discussed, is an illness that has a number of potential crisis points: the time of diagnosis; surgery; periods of chemotherapy or radiotherapy treatment; the start of remission; taking up the reins again; getting back to work; the threat or confirmation of recurrence; the periods of palliative treatment; and possibly the terminal stage of the illness and bereavement.

Each one of these potential crisis points provides its own challenge, and, having just come through one, you may have to face another almost immediately – and you can then feel as if you are on an emotional rollercoaster. Your flexibility and stamina will be your main strengths at these times.

Cancer in all its stages is a physical and emotional challenge for the patient, family, and friends. Your reactions are likely to be entirely consistent with those of people facing *any* enforced undesirable change. This particular challenge tests out your ability to come to terms with your own feelings in order to offer effective and constructive help. Your first instinct may be to find any way possible to escape what seems to be an overwhelming situation: to run away, to be anywhere rather than here. You will share, along with all those closely involved, periods of anger, frustration, helplessness, and depression. You will experience loss, periods of separation, and threats to your own security.

You can be forgiven if your first thought on hearing the diagnosis of cancer is 'what will become of me?' There is no reason to feel guilty about this, as it is quite a natural attitude when faced with the idea of losing someone. This may lead you to anticipate the death of your loved one, and emotionally go into mourning for everything that *could* be lost. At this point, you suffer a death of the spirit, and there is a real danger that you can 'write them off' emotionally. These reactions are shared by most who face this kind of crisis, and they are well documented.

When this happens, it is not easy to care for a sick person, to be positive, or to offer the kind of support needed. Your attempts to help may be clumsy at first, and this is only to be expected because you will be in the same state of shock as the person who has been diagnosed, be it partner, child, parent, brother, sister, or close friend. The illness threatens the security of everyone close to the patient. You are all under attack!

Some of you will accept the state of affairs quickly; some of you may deny it and try to carry on as though nothing has happened. You may even cope with your fears and anxieties by burying yourself in work that takes you away from the home; this serves to protect you from the full impact of the initial shock. You may find that the person diagnosed refuses to accept their condition, and makes it clear that no concessions will be made to the illness. However, the illness and its implications must be faced some time, and the sooner the better. In fact, people generally settle down and accept the true state of affairs within a period of four to six weeks.

## *Sorting things out*

The diagnosis is a highly emotional time, and many decisions are made without being thought through. The situation may demand a lot of activity and running around, and you may welcome this as a way of relieving anxiety. All this activity is happening while everyone is in a state of emotional turmoil and still coming to terms with the new situation. In these early stages of adjustment, decisions are made in a fragmented way; and as a result of anxiety and the feeling that our security is threatened, we may surprise ourselves at the way we react to minor irritations. You may even find that everyone around you is just as sensitive, and that anger may erupt in the form of bad temper and arguments. There may be unreasonable demands for attention at a time when no one is capable of providing it. We may blame others if things seem to be going wrong. This is the time for quiet discussion – be reassured that things will settle down as each one in turn finds their own way to accept the situation.

It is important for everyone to have the opportunity to talk about the way they feel so that ill-feeling isn't taken inside to fester and to continue to poison relationships. Discussion at this early stage can help set the tone for everyone to come together in a positive way as a team. After all, if you look at the situation calmly, you will appreciate that much of the emotion that we are feeling about the illness is being focused on to something else, usually trivial matters like whose turn it is to do the washing-up. The energy being wasted could be properly channelled to the benefit of the ill person and those most closely involved. If people feel encouraged in this way, then during the progress of the illness they may have the confidence to bring up problems as they arise.

## *Obligation and duty versus common sense –*
## *an offspring's obligations to parents*

If you are the son or daughter of the patient, you may – through a feeling of genuine concern and responsibility – feel that the only way you can manage your own family, and also have peace of mind about your parents, is to take them into your home. You may be an only child, and feel drawn by a sense of duty towards your parents, but before you rush into a far-reaching, irreversible decision, consider your own position. You may have children of your own who will still have to rely on you for physical and emotional support for a number of years. Are their needs likely to come into conflict with those of your parents? Can you cope with the stress of having to make frequent choices between your own family and your parents? Perhaps the work of caring will fall not on you, but on your partner. Can he or she cope? Will your health and your partnership take the strain? The decisions you have to make about the kind of support you can give are numerous, and these cannot be taken without full discussion that involves all members of the family – including those of your parents' own generation, perhaps their brothers or sisters.

Even if you live a long way away, there is a lot you can do to support your parents. What we are looking for is 'quality time' – frequent short visits can sometimes be enough to relieve the pressure and raise the spirits. Such visits are something to be looked forward to. In this way, relationships can remain intact because no one's independence is threatened. You may not be able to drop your own obligations – job, children, etc. – to be with your parents constantly, but it may be possible for you to be with them when things get really tough. Think about the crisis periods I have mentioned, and try to organize your visits and telephone calls around them. These are the times when you are really needed, even if it is just to do some hand-holding or provide some respite for the other parent who is carrying the workload. Your full-time presence may not be needed, unless in the short term the illness requires round-the-clock nursing.

Of course, not everyone will have the support of a team of

relatives and friends. Three-quarters of all people in this country who have cancer are elderly, and may be living alone or with an aged partner. If you find yourself in this situation, then you will be more dependent on outside help, both professional and voluntary. You may dearly wish to have the constant support of children who have long since left home, or who may have moved to distant parts. This can cause emotional turmoil for yourself and for your children, who may feel helpless and torn apart emotionally. You may have an expectation that children should do certain things for their parents, including giving up their home or offering you a home in times of trouble. Particularly vulnerable to this pressure are those adult female offspring who live on their own, and who may appear to have no good reason not to 'come back home'.

Or you as the patient may be under pressure to give up your home and move in with your son or daughter, and this idea may even be suggested or reinforced by some of your medical advisers. First, you should ask yourself whether you would have considered this option before the crisis of the illness. Would this be your first choice as a way to live? How well do you cope – apart from the illness? At this point, what kind of assistance do you think you really need, and can you get it from neighbours and friends or other local sources of help? Even in old age you must take a long-term view, and think about the advantages you gain from remaining independent in your own home, and in your own district, and weigh them against any possible short-term gains if you were to move away. Being a guest in someone else's home for a holiday is quite different from taking up permanent residence. Your children and their partners will have established quite a different lifestyle from your own, and if changes have to be made, it is you who will have to make them. A time of crisis is not the time to make such an important decision.

## *Obligation and duty versus common sense – troubled relationships*

It may be that you are in a marriage or relationship that has been strained for a long time before the onset of your partner's illness, or that the illness of your partner has been so testing of the relationship that you feel you have very little to offer. As a result, there may be guilt, leading you to over-compensate. This is not helpful to your partner, or to yourself. You may find that you are both locked into a situation where emotional blackmail and guilt characterize the relationship, and tension is constant. This is a time for honesty. Both of you have to consider the effects of this on each other and everyone around you.

If the atmosphere is constantly tense because of the relationship, then you and your partner may have to face up to the fact that progress towards health will be impeded. It will be obvious to your partner that your help is given grudgingly or with bad grace. He or she may feel happier being cared for by someone else, someone with whom they feel comfortable and more relaxed. If a relationship is bad, then a sick person will not want to feel under any obligation. It may be that a parting at this time would be extremely painful in the short term, and add to the stress of the illness. However, cancer can be a long-term illness, and your partner would have a better chance of recovery if parting resulted in the cause of the ever-present tension being removed. This may be a particularly important step to take in making lifestyle adjustments to ease stress during a remission period. My advice would be to talk matters over with a social worker or an organization such as Relate.

## Martyrdom has no place in caring

Everyone's situation is different, but no one is called upon to do *everything*. Many will try to do so, but at what cost? This is the stuff of 'martyrdom', but it does not guarantee that the patient is cared for adequately or that you and other family members are not being neglected in the process. It is no use 'caring' for one person at the expense of your own or anybody else's physical or mental health.

It is so easy to fall into the trap of 'martyrdom' during a period of acute illness or at the terminal stage. At this time, the person who is ill may cling to you and not want you to leave them alone. You may be able to sustain being tied this closely over a matter of some days, but when the days become weeks or even months, and everything else has been shelved, then it is obvious that your own needs and those of other people have also been put aside.

There may be times in a post-operative period, or on bad days, or in the terminal stage, when more constant attention is needed. However, when the illness is long term and has many different phases, there needs to be flexibility; and the patient is often the best judge of his or her own needs.

In the carer's mind, tender, loving care leads to people getting better, but this can be overdone. It is so easy to make someone feel powerless, with no control over many aspects of life. If the opportunity to do even the simple things such as washing, shaving, and fetching and carrying is denied, then it is easy to become helpless, acquiescent, and to sink into a decline. Obviously, this is not what the carer is aiming at. Good care involves encouragement to continue doing those things a fit person does as a matter of course. The aim is to ensure that capacity for independent action remains intact for as long as is physically possible. Sometimes it will be uncomfortable to stand by and watch slow progress in dressing and attending to personal hygiene, or moving about the house; it is so much easier to say 'Let me do that'. However, this denies the patient the opportunity to exercise responsibility, and emphasizes the 'sickness' aspect.

Those periods when extra care is needed are danger periods, and flexibility is important when these stages come to an end. This is the time to encourage a move towards normal living. Someone who is encouraged to be passive can respond to over-protective controlling care by regressing to 'babyhood', nurtured by the 'good parent'. This may be the easy way out for the person who does not want to upset the carer, or it may lead them to recognize their infantile position and to resent their state of helplessness. Heated exchanges may result that may bring about some adjustment in the situation, or establish an almost permanent battle for power.

Martyrdom can be forced on someone who is left to cope alone, being responsible for meeting all needs without anyone else's support. Because of this, it is very easy to become isolated from all other relationships. The 'martyr' has gone through a subtle psychological shift where nothing else appears to exist but the interdependence of them and their patient, together with a strong belief that no one else can do the job so well.

Everyone has a responsibility to guard against this happening to the principal carer. Thus it is extremely important for the family to see that this does not happen, and for visiting professionals to look out for the warning signs. The martyr may be extremely good at coping and covering up any signs that they are under stress: getting up very early to make the house presentable, doing all the washing, and preparing the patient for the daily round of visitors. The martyr may give the impression that they have everything under control, but it must be recognized by both professionals and family alike that it is not humanly possible for one person to bear the total workload of caring for a sick person. Sometimes the first and only indication that things are too much for such carers is a total, and seemingly sudden, collapse.

Caring is tiring, both physically and emotionally, and from time to time you will feel anger, frustration, irritability and depression. It is then that you will need someone to appreciate and understand this, and to be ready to move in with practical and emotional support. Your ability to go on caring without feeling martyred depends on this. No one enjoys being in the presence of a martyr who complains on the one hand, but will not accept help on the other.

## Asking for help

This can be difficult for many people. We live in a society where independence is encouraged at an early age, and we are judged on our ability to get on with the job in hand without grumbling. There are some who feel that only they can do a particular job properly; they are impatient with others, and are not prepared to wait for help to be offered. Or it may be that the help is offered, but turned down because the job cannot be done immediately. Many people are unhappy about asking for assistance because they feel it places them under some sort of obligation, and this makes them suspicious of offers of help. They have difficulty in accepting that help can be offered without any strings attached or thoughts of reward.

If you have difficulty in asking for help, then you too have to accept the premise that no one can care well for a sick person by themselves *and* come through the experience physically and emotionally intact. You have to accept that your own survival, and that of your loved one, may depend on your willingness to recognize that you need help – and to ask for it. Remember, it may be better for you to organize a number of people into carrying out some of the tasks, while you spend your precious time in conversation and enjoyable shared activities with your loved one. It may be the only time you have left to do it. Think constantly about your real priorities, and then put aside your reluctance to ask for the help that you need. Asking for help is not a sign of weakness – it is a sign of trust and maturity.

## Working together

As there are so many stages involved in cancer, it is important for all those who might be included in the team of helpers, as well as the patient, to have as much information from the professionals about what is required at each stage. Everyone should understand something of the nature of the patient's treatment and its purpose – for example, how long they are to be given a particular drug, its therapeutic benefits and side-effects, requirements following an operation, possible short-term or long-term disabilities, dietary requirements, frequency and duration of hospital visits, etc.

Before undertaking home nursing, it is as well to have as much information about the practical implications. Like many other people before me, I found myself learning as I went along. The most I had ever done previously was to lend a hand when the children had measles or act as nurse/cook during a family epidemic of flu. If lifting the patient is involved, then you are certainly going to need help. From personal experience, I can assure you that there is nothing worse than doing the job of caring in a state of uncertainty about the help available. Uncertainty makes people feel frightened, abandoned, and alone.

## Decisions about hospitalization or respite care

Coming to a decision about hospitalization can be extremely difficult for you. There will be times when, for medical reasons, there is no choice. Yet even when there is no choice, the idea of someone else caring for your loved one can be hard to take, especially if the doctor has come to the conclusion that you are exhausted and in no fit state to carry on. There can be a sense of guilt and failure that you are letting them down; your guilt may even be reinforced if other family members not so closely involved in day-to-day care insist it is your duty to carry on to the end. There are people who will not accept that anyone should be allowed to die away from their own bed; and when such people have these strong convictions, they often try to force them on to other people – and thus risk families being at war with themselves when all the energy is needed to cope with the anticipated loss and subsequent bereavement. If you look at this situation calmly, then it seems obvious that if you are caring intensively for someone who is seriously ill or dying, then you should be relieved of as much day-to-day care as possible in order that you can provide comfort to your loved one, and receive comfort yourself from other family members and friends.

The well-being of the patient can be threatened if the task of caring produces so much despair and anguish among family members that an atmosphere of negativity and depression pervades. There is a real prospect that the sick person suffers, and makes no progress. If the situation cannot be improved at home, then it may be that a hospice will provide a period of quiet supportive help and care – and experience shows that people admitted into hospice care actually flourish. They are no longer the source of worry and tension in the home. They no longer carry the burden of guilt for imposing strain on loved ones, and they are helped to engage with others in positive social contact. It is possible for many family wounds to be healed in an atmosphere of calm. No longer is there constant exposure to negativity; there is relief for patient and family alike. The growth of the hospice movement in recent years is an acknowledgement that people need a period of quiet supportive help and care at various stages during a long-term illness. (The idea of hospice care is discussed more fully in Chapter 8.)

## Who cares for the carer?

One of the most important tasks for family members and friends is to ensure the health and survival of the principal carers, those most closely involved in day-to-day care in the home. They should organize themselves to provide the principal carers with some respite, for carers can easily deteriorate in health as they skip meals, lose sleep, lose contact with friends, neglect themselves generally, and withdraw from social activities. They may be desperately worried about paying all the bills, which only adds to their anxiety. Expressions of concern from family and friends are not enough; the carers need to be looked after in as many practical ways as possible. Specifically, they need help with the day-to-day care of the patient, DIY jobs, gardening, shopping, etc. In particular, they need someone to come into the house to let them go out for a while to recharge their batteries. They even may need someone to take them out, and to help them get involved in things outside the sickroom. Someone coming in once every so often for a few hours to enable a woman to go to the hairdresser, etc., may do more to raise her spirits than a dozen phone calls. The irony is that visitors, without usually realizing it, put an added burden on the carer to provide hospitality.

# 8

# Sources of Support
## from Outside the Family

Many of the problems facing people during the crisis of cancer and other illnesses are practical ones; and if these problems are not dealt with, they can cause additional anxiety and worry. A number of these difficulties have already been touched on in previous chapters; and at this point I would like to bring together some information that you may find helpful.

## *Financial worries*

Long-term illness can lead to financial worries, and these worries can continue long after the illness is over. Most people who have serious prolonged illnesses or disabilities experience a reduction in their standard of living, and this is certainly no time to be proud. Explore every possible means of maintaining or supplementing your income via statutory and voluntary bodies, because the fewer changes you have to make in your living standards, the more you reduce stress from this area of your life. Unfortunately, membership of a private health scheme does not guarantee that you will receive financial help for a long-term illness; and if you are receiving private medical care, you may find that your benefits expire long before the treatment is completed. Illness imposes new and increased expenses – for example, travelling to and from hospital. Cancer treatment centres are few and far between, and can involve high travelling costs.

When a child has cancer, it may mean that one or both parents have to give up their jobs to look after them; and even when recovered, this child may remain dependent on the family long after the normal school-leaving period because they have problems in getting and keeping paid employment.

Rents, mortgages, and expenses for other services will still have to be met; and very often, when people are facing serious illness in their lives, these are the very things that are put to one side. Therefore it is very easy for arrears to build up. If you are already struggling to meet these expenses, then it is even more difficult when you have arrears. Administrators of these services are generally understanding if you can approach them when things *begin* to go wrong – don't wait until the bills have piled up! It is always possible to work out new and acceptable terms of payment. If you feel that in your present state you are not in the right frame of mind to negotiate these things for yourself, then seek help either from a medical social worker or the Citizens' Advice Bureau, or raise the matter with your doctor. In addition to national charities like the Malcolm Sargent Cancer Fund for Children, which gives help to meet children's needs, there are many other sources of income and practical help. Help may be allocated to meet specific needs – for example, transport. You might also explore with the local Lions, Round Table, or Rotary clubs what kind of help they can offer. They may not actually give you a financial gift, but they may offer practical help that will save you money.

## Work and employers

When cancer is diagnosed in an adult, it immediately throws into doubt their ability to carry on with their normal work. Ideally, the positive way to think about your illness is as an interruption in your working life, not an end to it. For this reason, it is important to try to put off any decision about giving up work for as long as possible. Certainly, do not think about making any decisions during the early days of the crisis; when people are in a state of shock, they do not think clearly. If they are undergoing treatment that undermines them both physically and emotionally, they are in no fit state to make far-reaching decisions.

This message is important for employers to be aware of, as well as patients and their families, and for this reason no one should be pressurized into making statements about when they expect to return to work, or about thinking of taking voluntary retirement. If there is any pressure at all, then immediately enlist the support of your doctor or consultant in writing to your employer to explain that you are not in a fit state to make a decision, and requesting them to be considerate. Some people have the decision to give up work forced upon them by employers, who quite legally can terminate their employment if the employee is unable to carry out their usual work or guarantee a return within a reasonably short period of time. It may be that you will think about continuing to work while you are having treatment. In this case, you will need an employer and colleagues who will tolerate your absence during treatment and recovery periods; they may have to accept that you can work only part-time, or reduce your normal work rate. Again, you may need to enlist the support of your medical advisers in your negotiations.

Generally, people are very generous in these circumstances. However, in order to accommodate the change in your work pattern, you may have to accept some reduction in income, particularly when your employer has to meet the increased cost of finding a part-time, temporary replacement. If your earnings do drop, you may perhaps qualify for Income Support, and your income tax and National Insurance contributions will be proportionally reduced.

## Education and schools

Children with cancer can often experience a prolonged interruption in their schooling. If they are fit enough, some education may be provided in hospital. When children return home, they may not always have the energy to follow a normal educational programme, and their illness may be such that they do not have the stamina or concentration to work at home. If you think there are likely to be problems about education, then by all means discuss with your local Education Department the possibility of the provision of home tutors. It may be that a home tutor for only a limited time during the day, say an hour or two, keeps alive the interest in education –but more than that, such visits can provide stimulation and encouragement, and symbolize that things are beginning to return to normal. During these difficult times, children can benefit from the experience of having a close, one-to-one relationship, and in fact learn very effectively.

If there is a possibility of your child returning to school, then let the head teacher know well in advance, because he or she will want to know the nature of your child's difficulties in order to assess the kind of help required. Arrangements may be made for part-time attendance at first, or for an auxiliary to assist your child in the practical problems of a school day. Don't expect your child to be able to sustain long periods of concentration or activity initially; these things take time. Children undoubtedly benefit from being with other children of their own age, and school is probably one of the best environments for re-establishing normal behaviour and contacts.

## Library service

Many people are unaware that local public libraries offer a mobile or home service to people who are housebound, and I found this to be a major lifeline for me during a prolonged illness. If you discuss your requirements with the library via the telephone you will probably be able to choose books, videos, and cassettes from the comfort of your own home.

## The value of groups to patients and carers

Fear is your enemy if you are coping with a long-term, and potentially life-threatening, illness. It uses up energy that is needed to support your body's fight against the illness; it also causes confusion, and can lead to depression and destructive thoughts.

You may be well supported at home, but because members of your family are coping with their own feelings and stress, their love may not be enough to help you through all the different stages of your illness and recovery – or you may not even have this support.

It may be that there are many practical and emotional issues that you have not been able to resolve. At this time, self-help or support groups are most important. Their members have been through it all – the anxieties, the tests, the diagnosis, treatments, adjustment to remission, perhaps bereavement, and the problems associated with reconstructing their lives. Together they have found the answers to many problems, and may still be finding answers to new ones.

Such groups can help you find and build on your inner strength to help you prepare for and meet many of the challenges of cancer. They are a fund of information about specific illnesses, treatments, and side-effects. They can provide access to practical and emotional help, boost self-esteem, help you back into social life, and reduce your sense of isolation.

Support groups have an overwhelming advantage over other forms of support in that they consist of people who have cancer and their families. Because of the common bonds within the group, people feel more relaxed and find it easier to communicate. Many people do not want to burden their family with all of their anxieties, and find it easier in broaching otherwise taboo topics of conversation with other cancer patients.

These groups can help people clarify thoughts that they may have trouble putting into words. This can be useful in formulating the right questions to put to doctors about all aspects of treatment and progress. When you belong to a group, you find that the help is two-way – and you will discover in time that you can offer as much to the group as you receive.

Many people fight shy of groups – they may never have been 'joiners' – and will need help in making the initial approach. To make this easier, POSY, a support group of parents of children with cancer at Yorkhill Hospital in Glasgow, man the library/rest room; here they can be available to parents during the crisis of their child's period in hospital. It is a place where parents can gain some respite from long vigils at the bedside, and find companionship and encouragement from others. This is a good way to introduce new people to the group. In this informal setting they can obtain information of various kinds, but the most important function is that they can get support when it is needed and feel the benefit of being with people sharing their experience. Positive feedback suggests that those who join in are less fearful, anxious, and depressed; and that they become more positive, and feel more at ease when talking about cancer. Some people will only need support from members of the group during the hospital stay. This is understandable, because this is a period of great anxiety.

The quality of the groups and their ability to help depends very much on the input of members and the experience and leadership capabilities of leaders. Groups do not usually offer formal therapy. Instead, they help people to find ways of coping that are useful to them. The most successful groups seems to be those that help people discover ways of adjusting to the illness and treatment, and lead people back into a satisfactory and rewarding life.

## *Varieties of support groups*

There are some groups that cater for people who share the same form of cancer or who have experienced similar treatment. For example, there are groups for women who have had mastectomies. They may include people who are qualified entirely by their own experience of self-help – or they may be trained patient volunteers, and offer individual counselling in addition to group support. Groups may include patients only, or open membership to patients and their families. They may be informal gatherings of a small number of people, e.g. a drop-in coffee morning or lunch group, or they can be more formally organized, involving patients, nurses, and doctors, and follow a programme of talks, discussions, and visits. Some may be entirely local, others may be affiliated to national organizations. The evidence suggests that people are more likely to join support and self-help groups when they terminate their treatment.

Studies carried out in the USA and Canada indicate that 'therapy' groups have a direct influence on survival. The suggestion is that people who adapt their lifestyle, emotional responses, and behaviour as a result of attending these groups will actually succeed in boosting their immune system. Research is currently being carried out to determine the precise influence of groups on prolonging and improving the quality of life. These groups are established either to run in parallel with medical treatment, or as a continuation of therapeutic help during remission periods. They are generally led by professionals qualified and experienced in helping people to work out for themselves new approaches to life – in other words, assistance is given to people who want to examine how they can adjust their lives to reduce stress. Such groups teach people strategies for coping with many situations, involving relationships and communication, that have hitherto caused them problems. There is a focus on building self-esteem and self-confidence, and developing ways to think and behave positively.

There are some parallels between such cancer groups in the USA and those run in the UK for helping people to manage their pain. All involve a process of education that entails strengthening the individual physically and emotionally, resulting in the ability to live more satisfactory and rewarding lives. My feeling is that resources, both financial and human, which are at present spread very thinly over a range of separate *ad hoc* groups, could be put to better use in establishing a more formal network of 'educational/therapeutic' groups. If this were to happen, then the undoubted power of people to help one another would be harnessed much more effectively.

## Professional carers

### Social workers

Every hospital has a social work unit staffed by trained people experienced in helping with all kinds of problems related to individuals and families. The purpose of social work help is to ensure that people are enabled to carry on functioning to the best of their ability while they or a member of their family have an illness. They are valuable sources of information and advice on financial matters, including benefits and grants that might assist towards general living costs, and the inevitable additional costs that accompany serious illness. It is possible to receive assistance with transport, particularly where children are involved, and to receive assistance with the provision of special diets, respite care, and practical aids. Mistakenly, many people see this as the only function of the social work department.

Social workers are also trained and skilled in assessing emotional needs, and they possess skills as counsellors. If something is troubling you, it is better to go and talk it over with someone – get it off your chest at an early stage. If you don't, your cause for concern may interfere with the medical treatment for cancer being given to you or a member of your family. The social worker will also be able to judge whether or not you need more specialist help with an emotional problem such as depression or anxiety. It is unfortunate that to many of the general public, social work help has become synonymous with help given to the poor; and a misplaced sense of pride prevents some families from seeking social work help when this might be appropriate. The social work department is there for *everybody* in crisis who feels the need for help. You do not need to go through a doctor or a nurse to get the help; you can refer yourself directly to the social work office in the hospital.

A recent development has involved the appointment of social workers responsible for following through with home visits to children and families after they have left hospital. It has been recognized that many families feel isolated after a child has left hospital, and that many emotional and behavioural difficulties can be eased by social work intervention. This initiative is being backed with financial help from the Malcolm Sargent Cancer Fund for Children. Social workers can also be helpful to individuals and families coming to terms with the diagnosis of cancer, or the realization that their particular illness is terminal, and in cases of bereavement.

### The clinical psychologist

Referral to a clinical psychologist may be made through your hospital consultant, your family doctor, or the hospital social worker. The clinical psychologist is trained, as the name suggests, in all matters relating to the psychology of illness. Many people need positive help when they are suffering from a depressive illness; such illness may result from traumatic experiences within the family, as a result of your medical treatment, bereavement, or exhaustion through taking on too much without adequate support – particularly if you are caring for a sick person. If you are the patient, it may be that the clinical psychologist will be part of the team responsible for helping you manage your pain. There are many skills and techniques that psychologists can help with that will make life more comfortable. There is no shame in having the help of the psychologist, who is just one of a team of specialists in any hospital. Anybody who is ill, or who has a member of the family seriously ill, is involved emotionally as well as physically. The psychologist is there to ensure that your emotional and psychological health is taken care of, and that it does not interfere with your ability to cope with the illness and with life in general.

### Community nurse

The community nurse (district nurse) is usually the main provider of practical nursing care within the home, and your doctor or hospital will make arrangements for the kind of tasks they need to carry out. It may be that you will need help with dressings, bathing, or advice on medication and diet to overcome specific problems as they arise. Community nurses are an important link between the family and your doctor, and they will ask him to visit you if this is necessary. Because they are so intimately involved with patients and families, they are in an ideal position to reassure, give a sense of proportion, and to provide immediate emotional support.

### Macmillan nurse

Macmillan nurses are specifically trained to undertake all aspects of nursing care associated with cancer. Some are attached to hospitals or hospital districts, and are available for consultation and advice from the time of diagnosis. They have detailed knowledge of individual forms of cancer and its care, and are trained to understand and deal with the emotional aspects of the illness. They can also provide valuable help to patients and their families during the illness and, if necessary, during a period of bereavement. In many cases, they can ease the communication between patients and consultants, and will readily explain precisely what is involved in the various aspects of treatment. You can refer yourself directly to a Macmillan nurse if there is one in the hospital you are attending. Don't be put off by a consultant who says they will be available 'when you need them . . .'. It is not intended that Macmillan nurses appear only at a terminal stage – they can help at any point during your illness. From information obtained when I was researching this book, I know that they *prefer* to be involved with the patient at the time of diagnosis – if this is requested. Although the value of Macmillan nurses is increasingly recognized, there are still too few of them to meet the need.

### Marie Curie nurse

If you are being nursed at home, it is often possible to call upon the services of a Marie Curie nurse via your GP or community nurse when your carers require assistance, particularly during the night. This is of great benefit to carers who have to carry on caring during the day. It enables them to relax and have an undisturbed night's sleep, knowing that their loved one is in good hands.

### Hospice care

Hospices specialize in providing terminal or respite care. Sometimes the burden of caring in the home is too great for people who are old or infirm themselves, or if there is not sufficient family support. Families who have been caring for someone for a long time may simply be worn out and need a respite, and can be helped by the patient's admission to a hospice. A hospice specializes in providing high-quality nursing care that takes into account the emotional and spiritual needs of the patients and their families. The hospice is not subject to the normal emergency demands of a general hospital, and so the environment is more peaceful and the surroundings are specially designed to provide a homely atmosphere. When patients are admitted to hospices, they often find that they achieve a higher quality of life than they have for some time, for particular consideration is given to reducing and controlling pain and discomfort.

In recent years, some hospices have been able to send out staff into the community to provide a specialized nursing service that gives the same quality of care as that received in the hospice. This form of care supplements the work of the community nurses.

### Complementary therapists

It is not within the scope of this book to explore the advantages of using complementary therapists as a substitute for traditional medicine. Complementary therapists skilled in such things as acupuncture, massage, reflexology, hypnotherapy, psychotherapy, herbalism, naturopathy, and spiritual healing can all offer something of value to the cancer sufferer at various times. The individual professional associations can provide information about the specific services they offer, and will indicate the names and addresses of people approved by them to practise. It is very important that you approach the individual professional bodies or the British Institute of Complementary Medicine, or your own doctor, for advice on whom to approach – *never* call on the services of anyone who claims that they can cure cancer. It is illegal to make such claims, and anyone who does is unlikely to be recognized as fit to practise. The main purpose of seeking complementary help would be to augment, and not to replace, your medical care. Practitioners can certainly help you to feel more comfortable physically, reduce your anxiety, raise your spirits and, as a result, enable you to cope with cancer more successfully.

# 9
## Dealing with Sadness

This chapter is about the way in which members of families can combine to support one another in their efforts to cope with periods of sadness as a result of cancer. It is not easy, and demands a high degree of commitment and flexibility from everyone concerned. It doesn't just happen!

In the introduction to this book, I talked about the strong emotional links in a family, and the feelings – sometimes positive, sometimes negative – that characterize family relationships. Families go through many experiences together, and on the whole the family unit provides every member with enough security and support to survive and function through both good and bad periods. However, there is a lot of evidence that shows that as well as a high degree of positive feeling between family members, there is likely to be an almost equal amount of negative feeling. Love can be experienced very strongly – but so can hate. If you were brought up with a number of brothers and sisters, you can probably remember the intensity of feeling that you experienced from time to time; but because people in a family live so closely together, they usually learn to appreciate each other's likes and dislikes – the things that produce happiness, the things that produce sadness or anger. They accommodate to each other's periods of ill-health, depression, rebellion, and thoughtlessness, and develop ways of bringing erring members back into line. At its best, the family unit is able to provide for a diverse group of personalities of all ages, enabling them to develop as individuals pursuing their own goals, even when they live away from the family home.

When someone has a life-threatening or long-term illness that substantially changes their ability to function alone, the family is called upon to provide care and support over and above the normal levels. The progress of such illnesses calls for many adjustments to be made, and they are a real test of the strength of the family. The family has to cope with the fact that an otherwise outgoing member may have long periods when they are morose and withdrawn, or a calm person becomes short-tempered. Other members have to adjust to the fact that the strongest, most competent, member might become helpless and dependent. Roles change, workloads alter, and each member may be called upon to make sacrifices in time, money, leisure activity, or even professional ambition. When these adjustments take place, they may provoke strong feelings of fear, disappointment, anger, injustice, and guilt. Once recognized, these problems need to be brought out into the open so that they are not suppressed and allowed to fester. With the interests of the patient being foremost, new ways of coping can be explored, and agreement reached on how best to reconcile everyone's needs. Caring means sharing responsibility.

In spite of the best intentions of family members, there are times when one member takes on major responsibilities – or has them forced upon him or her. It may be that one person is extremely sensitive to the climate of feeling around them, and consciously or unconsciously takes on responsibility for 'tension management' within the family.

When things are going well, this person may be able to jolly people along or guide their attention away from their problems. You have probably seen a mother deal with a sulking child by diverting their attention to a fresh, exciting activity. Sometimes this works, sometimes not – and several tries may be needed before the child chooses to do something positive (or, in desperation, needs to be disciplined). Some of us can be aware that someone is feeling upset, disturbed, or sad, and patiently wait for the mood to change. Others take the matter personally, and set out to change the climate of feeling. Anyone caring for someone with cancer is likely to be confronted by that person's suffering – which may be expressed as anger, irritability, anxiety, frustration, or sadness – and the carer can feel a personal responsibility for easing the suffering.

## 'I'll cry if I need to . . .'

Anyone who has to live closely with someone who suffers is torn apart emotionally by the fact that they are helpless to bring about an immediate change for the better. However, carers need to guard against being over-sensitive to looks, words, or behaviour – or even believing that they personally are causing the patient to feel sad, depressed, or irritable. It is easy to forget that from time to time all of us feel sad at the loss of one thing or another, although of course these feelings are likely to occur more frequently and more intensely when coping with a serious long-term illness. As a result, as a carer you may attempt to change the emotional climate by trying too hard to find ways to 'make up' for your own imagined lack of sensitivity. This, of course, is a complete misunderstanding of the situation, and if the desired change in mood does not take place, then you can be left confused, hurt, and even more helpless.

It is hard to live with someone who is going through a period of sadness, but you have to allow an opportunity for these feelings to be worked through, or shared in due course. The patient may feel remorse at having displeased the carer by his or her lack of response. The result may be deeper depression on the one hand, and feelings of frustration and inadequacy on the other. If the situation continues, then there is the danger of an enormous barrier in communication.

Take the following example. John was in a period of remission following several months of treatment for leukaemia. After two months at home, he had clearly demonstrated that he was ready to begin work again for his school-leaving examinations. His disposition was normally sunny and he was popular, but from time to time he would retire to his room to lounge for hours on his bed listening to records. This normal teenage behaviour made his mother feel very uncomfortable, and whenever it happened she bombarded him with suggestions that he phone a friend, invite someone round, anything but shut himself away. He generally responded angrily or simply ignored her. Because of his illness and her genuine concern, John's mother could not accept John's behaviour as normal for his age and situation. Instead, she felt she might have upset him or, even worse, that his illness might be worrying him – as well it might. In desperation, she constantly interrupted his self-imposed isolation with enquiries about whether he was all right – could she get him anything? Should she invite someone round to keep him company and cheer him up? And then, as her frustration at her inability to get through to him increased, she berated him for not studying, for not making an effort, and so on.

John's mother had taken responsibility for his feelings, and tried to change them. From time to time, all of us feel low, sad, or irritable, and need to be on our own – we need this space to come to terms with our present situation before moving on. It is not helpful to 'programme' anyone out of the way they feel by 'jollying them along'. In fact, John's mother was denying him the right to feel sadness, or any other emotion, unless she approved of it! Everyone needs time to come to terms with loss, to experience a period of sadness before moving on. In this respect, John was like Maureen – whom we met in Chapter 4 – in that he resisted attempts to have 'his strings pulled'.

## When someone is terminally ill

The prospect of someone dying highlights relationships within the family, and forces everyone to face the prospect of change; and this, of course, is very frightening. Sadness is not the only feeling aroused at this time. Instead, it may sometimes seem as if anger is the predominant emotion. As carer, you are faced with your own impotence, and in frustration you may express your anger towards the person who is ill. The prospect of their dying causes you to anticipate your own loss. You may be angry with them because they do not appear to be fighting it – it may seem as if they have accepted the inevitable. Teenagers, particularly, confronted by a dying parent and experiencing confusion, bewilderment, and fear, combined with an intense feeling of anger at their own situation, may need to escape from the 'hothouse' – and may even leave home, seeking some relief in the company of other youngsters in a normal teenage environment. Even here, though, they may find themselves alienated, because no one else can share their experience. This period of anticipatory grief can be overwhelming, and all the attention at this stage is focused on the person who is ill. Outbursts of anger on the part of close family members may be ways in which they convey that they are also suffering, and need some help and support to cope with what seems to them an impossible situation.

Waiting for someone to die can seem like a marathon; a period of prolonged uncertainty. It is a time when all other aspects of life are suspended. There may even be feelings that the sick person should die quickly in order to put an end to everybody's suffering, and so that they can get on with life. Everyone involved in caring will feel an urgent need to escape from the situation. This is a time when the family must come together and share the burdens, and to support one another. It is a time when everyone has intense feelings, and things may be said that hurt and cause irreparable damage to family relationships. It is a time, therefore, for everyone to recognize this, and to make allowances and be forgiving.

There is much evidence to suggest that, whether or not they are undergoing crisis, families ensure their survival as a unit by displacing their bad feelings. These bad feelings of anger, fear, and guilt can be directed outwards, and families will unite in enmity towards officialdom, neighbours, or other families to preserve their common identity. Although the targets of such feelings can often be left feeling bruised and bewildered, the family members themselves can feel strengthened. Ultimately, however, these attacks on people outside the family may serve to cut off or limit sources of valuable help.

Sometimes families turn their feelings against one of their own number. They 'elect' a scapegoat to carry all the bad feelings and the blame for everything that is going wrong. In times of crisis, when feelings are running very high, the unfortunate scapegoat – who is unable to do anything right in the eyes of the family – will be carrying an intolerable burden, particularly if the scapegoat is a child already weighed down with personal anxieties and fears. There is a real risk that the physical and emotional health of the scapegoat will suffer, and in the end the whole family may be threatened with disintegration. Obviously, this helps no one.

The intensity of feelings at this time may be so great that there is an attempt to exclude children, teenagers, or more delicate family members from experiencing fully all that is involved in the terminal stage of the illness. Anyone who is excluded in this way will feel unimportant and left out. This exclusion can be experienced as a loss, and may later add to the sadness and emptiness that is involved in the grief following a death. It can contribute to grief remaining unresolved, leaving the person confused and depressed. Everyone needs to be able to make the choice for themselves about the part they play during this terminal stage. The terminal stage should be a signal for the family to come together to ensure that the dying person experiences as many positive ways as possible of connecting to family and friends.

## *Keeping pace with one another*

During a check-up following an operation, Bryan was informed that his cancer could have spread and that further investigations would be needed to determine the extent before deciding on whether it would be possible to offer further treatment. Believing up till then that all the cancer had been successfully removed, Bryan was plunged into dismay and depression, and all the fears about his survival returned. Unfortunately, the tests confirmed the suspicion, and he was told that over the next few months he would steadily deteriorate. He was told not to worry about it now . . . the hospital would arrange for visits from the district nurse and the Macmillan nurse, who would see that he was kept pain-free and comfortable. Suddenly, the situation had changed from one of looking forward to recovery, to one of hopelessness. While in this shocked state, he asked for details of what to expect in the terminal stage, and he was given a comprehensive 'countdown' of the next six months. Within two days of returning home, he received a form to complete for attendance allowance. The heading invited the applicant who had less than six months to live, to complete, sign, and return the form, countersigned by their doctor. To Bryan, this was confirmation that the death sentence had been passed.

Bryan had always been a philosophical man, and having reached his mid-seventies he had been reconciled to the idea of dying. What he found hard to take was this all-too-honest, almost business-like approach. Up to this point he had been feeling well, spent a couple of hours each day in the garden, took his dog out two or three times a day, took Janet, his wife, out in the car, went shopping, and carried on doing the usual sort of odd-jobs around the home. He had very little discomfort, though he had lost some weight. The prognosis was hard to believe, and Bryan at first responded by denying that the doctors could be right about this. As the news sank in, though, he became very depressed, and lost interest in all those activities that he was physically able to do.

Janet had a strong sense of duty, and had always been concerned that no one should have cause to criticize the way she cared for her family. Her love was expressed in the quality and quantity of food on the table, the cleanliness of the house, and the hospitality provided to visitors. Throughout her life she had responded to loss and difficulty by soldiering on, always showing a brave face to the world. The emotion she found easiest to express was anger and rage at the unfairness of life, and the incompetence of others 'who ought to know better'.

Bryan was by this stage housebound, and found himself spending longer and longer each day alone with his own feelings as his wife kept herself continually busy in the kitchen for long stretches. These periods in the kitchen were being used to brood on her problems, and from time to time she would emerge, using a wooden spoon to emphasize certain points that gave vent to her feelings about the unreliability of doctors' visits, the delays experienced when visiting hospital, the rudeness of the hospital staff, and the stupidity of the visiting nurse getting into detailed discussions with her husband about his illness, and so forth. Her main theme was that medical staff in general had very little understanding of people. 'Fancy giving him all that information all at once. They were far too blunt. And then to let him just walk out and drive home along that busy motorway – he might've killed us both!'

Bryan's sense of isolation and despair increased. Janet was still so angry, having been confronted with the worst possible news, that she was beyond being comforted – and was in no position to offer comfort to Bryan. She could not handle his deterioration, and called upon Bryan's brother Tom – who had always had a close relationship with him – to come and spend a few days with them. Tom readily agreed, and came straight away. Janet took his coming as an opportunity to use him as an audience for all the comments that she wanted to make about the professional carers involved in Bryan's case. Tom was given a blow-by-blow account (several times over) of the history of Bryan's illness and its treatment since its inception, even though he was already well informed about everything that had gone before. Bryan was portrayed as the innocent victim of an inadequate health service, and he sat through all of this passively hour after hour.

What they both really needed at this time was a period of calm. Bryan had actually fully accepted the situation and needed a period of reflection, and, as he said later, he was looking for someone to reassure him that he would be able to face death with dignity and without pain. He also wanted reassurance that Janet would not be overwhelmed with the physical task of caring for him.

Janet had not reached this stage of acceptance. She was feeling bruised, her anger was still very strong, and beneath this anger was a natural fear about coping with Bryan's death, and what her life would be like afterwards. She was going through a period of anticipatory loss, hence the strong feelings. It was easier to blame others for her pain at this stage; and of course the way in which the situation had been handled added fuel to her strong feelings, and made it difficult for her to work through them and resolve them.

Tom was patient, and when eventually Janet had exhausted her tirade he encouraged his brother to unload his worries. Initially, Janet retreated to the kitchen, but after a few minutes would interrupt the conversation with offers of refreshment, asking what they would like for lunch, asking if they were warm enough, or cutting across their conversation by directly questioning Tom about his own family. For Janet, it seemed dangerous to discuss anything more than trivia.

It was only by prolonging Tom's stay and making the best of their opportunities that Tom and Bryan were able to open up a channel that would allow the expression of feelings, fears, and worries. This channel was effective, and Bryan perked up and began to take an increased interest in life and to prepare for the next stage of his illness. In fact, having got things off his chest, he recognized that he could make positive use of his remaining time; and by the day that Tom returned home, he had resumed his full range of activities – even taking Tom down to the local. As Bryan became more settled and more active, Janet visibly relaxed, and began to enjoy once more the things they had done together.

The two brothers continued to keep in touch by telephone, but whenever Tom phoned, Janet – who had taken to answering all incoming calls – would give him all the details of Bryan's progress until there seemed no more questions he could ask. Eventually Tom persisted that he wanted to speak directly to his brother, and only then was the phone handed over – with reluctance. Although Bryan had fully accepted his situation, Janet still wanted to deny the reality, and placed herself between her husband and everyone else – including the nurses with whom he might wish to discuss anything connected with his health. She was happy as long as he was carrying on normally; she did not want to be reminded of his deteriorating condition.

Janet's reaction is a perfectly normal one in the situation. It is common at the terminal stage for people who are close to the situation to come to terms with the prospect of death in quite different ways and at different speeds. The dying person often accepts the situation more quickly and with more equanimity. They want to be reassured about the nature of death; and they are concerned, too, that those they leave behind will be all right. The last thing that those close to them want to accept is that death is approaching; they have their own fears about losing a loved one and about surviving alone. It is a frightening prospect, and, because of this, Bryan was looking to other people to help him prepare for it in the most sensitive way possible. Janet was distracting herself by following a routine of cooking and other familiar activities – perhaps as reassurance that nothing is changing. In spite of this apparent denial, Janet came to terms with the situation in her own time.

Anxiety and fear can be dealt with by following familiar routines; this allows time for equilibrium to be restored and is valuable preparation for facing a new and difficult situation.

Bryan's remaining few months were very positive, and during this time he planted out his garden with a range of plants that would flower the whole year round. Each day he and Janet made time to listen to their favourite music and enjoy their shared love of poetry reading. Eventually, both arrived at the same point, acknowledging that when you have lived for almost eighty years, you have enjoyed and shared many rich experiences – and death is part of this.

In families, the idea that a loved one is dying is not accepted by everyone at the same time. The idea can be so frightening to some that there is no acceptance, but constant denial of the real situation, and this can make coming to terms much more protracted. When the terminal cancer sufferer is a child, it is often the mother who faces up to the situation earlier than the father – this is particularly so when he goes out to work. The fact of the child's illness and possibility of death is constantly with the mother. She is carrying out all the practical aspects of care, and has more opportunity to discuss progress with medical staff. When the father is working, away from the home or hospital environment, he has to 'switch off' if he is to concentrate on his job. The mother, realizing the pressure on the father, may even protect him from the full impact of the child's illness – and unconsciously establish a pretence that things are not as bad as they really are, and that she can cope while he goes to work. The realization of the severity of the cancer, when it finally comes, can be completely devastating, and hospital social workers are often called upon to help parents cope with the strong emotions aroused at this time. There may be feelings on the part of the father that things have been kept from him; he may even feel angry towards his wife for her part in a 'conspiracy with the doctors'.

These feelings need to be coped with as both parents have their role to play with their sick child, and at the terminal stage it is not helpful to have parents pulling in opposite directions. At this point, there is a need for both parents to talk and acknowledge their fears to each other. It is a time to find out about the progress of the illness, and to make practical decisions about informing the family, the possibility of home or hospital care, the care of other children in the home, and making use of the remaining time in the most positive way. How much you tell the sick child depends on a number of things: the age, and the level of understanding and preparedness.

Some children are well aware of the progress of their illness and of the possibility of death. They may have many questions to ask about the nature of death, and the way in which they will die. These questions are often posed by healthy children out of natural curiosity. However, a sick child may hold back from asking these kinds of questions for fear of upsetting the parents. The child may, in fact, pretend that things are better than they are. One mother I talked to said, 'No matter what I've been told or how I'm feeling, I make a point of going into the ward with a broad smile on my face and keep it there – fixed – throughout the visiting time. This is a terrific strain, but I don't want him to see I'm sad or worried.' Both parents and children may need help in putting aside their pretences.

At any stage in the illness, parents can become overwhelmed by their own anxiety and fear that their child might die; and even when a child is undergoing treatment or has entered a period of remission, they hold on to their anxiety, unable to accept any good news. They may persist with their feeling that they should prepare themselves and their child in the event that death will be the eventual result. I met one parent who was very upset that she had initially allowed her anxiety to influence her, and she had then spent some days reading with her child a series of booklets designed to help children face the prospect of dying. She suddenly realized that in fact her child was making good progress, and that the material she was asking the child to dwell on was not relevant to the situation.

As at any other time, it is important to be sensitive to where your child is in the process of acceptance. It means allowing an opportunity for questions to be asked and, when they come, to answer them honestly. All parents will know that the most profound questions come quite naturally and out of the blue, perhaps during a game or drawing pictures. In a family that already has a climate of sharing and involving children in discussions about family affairs, there are unlikely to be many secrets. It is unfortunate if the child is holding on to a secret and thinks the parents are not ready to hear it, or, if the parents and family are keeping secrets. When this happens, everyone remains isolated, and in no position to help one another.

## Bereavement and loss

Many people who have cared for a loved one during a long illness that terminates in death will experience a sense of relief. It can feel as though a burden has been lifted – not a physical burden, but a release from all that is associated with confinement in a sickroom: the waiting, the uncertainty, the anguish, the exhaustion, the lack of sleep. At last you too are being let out from the confinement of the sickroom. Sometimes it can even feel like a sense of elation, but this is no reason to feel guilty. This emotion is real, and it is part of the normal reaction of coming through an extremely difficult period – you have survived! This feeling of elation probably won't last, though. There will be tears, feelings of loss, and you will go through the normal process of grieving, and experience a sadness that may last for many months. You may feel your grief very intensely. It may seem as though there is nothing left for you, that nothing good will ever happen again, that it's all in the past. These feelings have to be worked through, even if they are very painful. Your sadness and loneliness may be increased by feelings of anger, resentment, and guilt.

You may find yourself idealizing the one who has died, perhaps even creating a shrine to their memory – either physically or within your own mind. However, you will work through all these feelings, and the time will come when it is possible to begin to look forward to a life without that person: to enjoy new experiences, new ventures, new places. Some people feel very guilty about starting new things, even when they are ready to do so, because of some mistaken belief that they will always be tied to that person. But remember, beginning again is healthy, and does nothing to betray the quality of life you had with that person, or destroy their memory.

There are things that make grieving difficult: the amount of change that is forced on you as a result of the death, your physical ability to make changes, and the strength of the emotion you were experiencing during the final days and weeks. You may have been through a very difficult period with other people at this time, and there may be a lot of anger and resentment about this that has never been properly dealt with. You may also have regrets that you were unable to put certain things into words to your loved one before they died, which might have had the effect of resolving issues that were outstanding between you.

You might find it helpful to close your eyes for a moment and resolve things now . . . Just imagine yourself saying those things that were left unsaid – you may even want to say them out loud. They may not always be pleasant things, but whatever you say, say it with whatever emotion feels real for you.

## *Children need special treatment*

When an older person dies, we often comfort ourselves by celebrating their life and remembering the years they have enjoyed with their family. When a child dies, it seems so much more of a tragedy, because so much remains unfulfilled. What seems so unfair is that a child's life has barely got started, that talents have remained undeveloped, and that there has been so little time to share with them. Many people losing a child speak of the loss leaving them with a permanent feeling of emptiness, with a gap in their lives that can never be filled. The creativity of parenthood, beginning with the conception of the child and culminating in independence, has been cut short. Child-rearing is a fundamental task; and when it is left incomplete, it is little wonder that parents feel as though they have lost part of themselves. Other children in the family and any later children will never be substitutes for the one who has died. Each child has a value of its own and is special.

Unfortunately, a sick and dying child does take away so much energy and time from the healthy children in the family that the latter can feel neglected, confused, and angry that for a time they must take a back seat. Grieving parents can be so absorbed in their own loss that they fail to recognize the importance of the loss to their other children, who experience all their feelings of bereavement from an immature point of view. They will experience not only their own sadness at the loss of a brother or sister, but a sadness at the feeling that their parents have turned away from them. It is difficult to grieve *and* still have time, energy, and emotional strength to give to others – yet this is what is demanded of parents. They need help to do this. They need to be relieved of as many day-to-day pressures as possible, so that they can begin to rebuild relationships with their remaining children.

When parents continue for a long time in their grief and talk of nothing else but the lost child and their feeling that nothing can ever replace that child, the other children can feel that they are of lesser value, and somehow ought to be filling the gap left by the dead child. Children will not necessarily have the words to talk about this, and their grieving, confusion, and depression may be expressed in withdrawal, bad behaviour, poor schoolwork, or other symptomatic behaviour such as bed-wetting, truancy, defiance, or even delinquency. While the parents are absorbed in their grief, it may be that aunts, uncles, grandparents, or friends recognize the suffering of the children and allow them to experience what it means to be special. It doesn't mean heaping them with gifts as a substitute for their loss – it means giving generously of time and energy, and showing a willingness to listen in order to help the child come to terms with the momentous things that have been happening. The whole family has to accept responsibility for healing this grief, and helping the most vulnerable members to regain their confidence and self-esteem.

## *Sometimes grief is not fully resolved*

You will see from the following story that a lot of adjustment was needed as a result of Reg's death. Lorna, his wife, had fundamental changes to make. Her position was complicated by the strong feelings that overwhelmed her immediately before and after his death, and her grieving process was disrupted by these emotions.

This is a story of a couple living and working on the Costa del Sol. Reg had been a golf professional, who had achieved moderate success in his early years. When this part of Spain began to be developed for tourism and leisure complexes were built, Reg was offered a job as the golf professional at one of them, but after about three years he took over as General Manager, responsible for running the whole complex. For 15 years Lorna and Reg lived in what might be said to be a state of luxury in idyllic surroundings. He was well paid, ran a Mercedes, and the couple were well known as generous hosts and party-givers. Lorna had no specific role to play, except as 'consort' to her husband, but like many other wives she provided a strong emotional base for Reg. Her life was devoted to his welfare. Her only independent activity was as a member of the theatre club attached to a small theatre based in a town 20 miles away, run for and by British ex-pats. She enjoyed the exchange of reminiscences of how life used to be in Britain.

Occasionally, the couple visited their elderly parents in the Manchester area. More often than not, their parents came out to stay with them for two or three months at a time, relishing the warm climate. To all intents and purposes, Reg and Lorna had lost touch with other family and friends in England.

When he was 48, Reg began to feel unwell, but because he was in the middle of a busy season he tended to disregard the symptoms he was experiencing. He put off consulting a doctor, thinking that he would combine a consultation with his routine annual medical at company headquarters in London. Lorna was extremely anxious about him, and was upset that he would not listen to her pleas for him to see a doctor locally. By the time of the trip, he looked ill and was easily tired. On arrival in London, the company doctor carried out his examination and arranged for him to be admitted to hospital immediately for further tests; but before the tests were completed, Reg was put on morphine. He had only been in the hospital two days! Frantically, Lorna set about seeking further information. No one at the hospital would tell her anything other than, 'We are still awaiting the results of the tests.' The company doctor attempted to reassure her, saying, 'Reg is in the best hands, and getting the best attention. Just be patient.'

Lorna moved into a small hotel near the hospital so that she could be near Reg. Each day she sat in the ward for hours on end, trying to find out from the staff what was happening. The staff kept repeating that they were still awaiting results of the tests, and that until these came through they could not commit themselves. On the third day, when the consultant visited Reg, she was asked to wait outside in the corridor. She asked the ward sister if she could speak to the consultant after the examination. The corridor was crowded because it was visiting time; children were running up and down, playing. After what seemed hours, the consultant came out to her, and in this public area informed her that her husband had an untreatable liver cancer, and that it was just a matter of time . . .

This was Lorna's first indication that Reg's illness was cancer, and before she had a chance to take in this news, she was overwhelmed by the further revelation that it was terminal. In fact, he lived for only another six weeks.

The problems affecting Lorna were numerous. First of all, she felt completely isolated; there was no one near that she could talk to. This was a crisis of major proportions. Fear about her husband's condition had been made intolerable by her inability to obtain basic information about his condition. Her natural anxiety was not recognized, and she felt completely cut off by the stone-walling attitude of the staff at the hospital. The way she was eventually informed was, to her, brutally insensitive. She was left by the consultant, in tears in the crowded corridor, too stunned to move. There was no one there to comfort her, and she was in no state to offer any solace to her husband at that stage. She was left to face the loneliness of her hotel room, and to phone Reg's father and her own parents to break the news. They were equally stunned by the sudden turn of events.

More than anything, she felt helpless to change the situation and felt guilty. She swore that had their roles been reversed, her husband would have moved heaven and earth to prevent her from dying – and she really believed this. He had been the strong one and organizer of their life together. She knew this idea was quite irrational and that in reality nothing she had done would have saved Reg. She knew also that had the situation been reversed Reg would have been equally powerless. Even though she accepted her belief as irrational, it was not enough to remove her sense of guilt.

This kind of sudden change can happen as a result of any one of a number of events such as a stroke, heart attack, or accident. Even the threat of such events can trigger off anxiety, and cause us to anticipate loss. In this case, it was cancer that brought about a complete change in lifestyle. In the initial period of shock, Lorna was overwhelmed by the loss of her husband. Gradually, as she emerged from this shock, she began to realize how his death had completely changed everything. Their luxury home went with the job, and that meant finding somewhere else to live immediately. Someone else would have to be appointed to Reg's job, so it would be impossible for her to return to her old lifestyle in the complex. Her position as hostess had gone, and she realized that she had no close friends there – they were merely acquaintances. After 15 years, that life had gone for ever, and she could not see any reason to return to Spain.

Therefore in Lorna's case, mourning was related to even more than the loss of her lifelong partner. Even five years after his death, she still feels she is drifting. In spite of being highly intelligent, possessing many social skills, and still only in her forties, she has been unable to plan for a life as a single person. She is still hurting, and focuses her pain specifically on her perception of the insensitive, offhand manner of the consultant who gave her the news. She still relives that scene in the corridor. So far, she has been unable to put that behind her, and to employ her undoubted ability to rebuild her life; but she is making a start by recognizing that others are probably going through the same experiences and have the same feelings of helplessless, guilt, and despair. She is tryng, through a voluntary organization, to be available to offer emotional and practical help at the time of diagnosis. Thus far, her own emotional needs have been put to one side; she feels she would be letting her husband down if she did anything that smacked of seeking pleasure or happiness for herself. Everything she does must be for a 'good cause' – but she does not see herself as a 'good cause'.

Putting grieving behind you and accepting fully your new situation means that you recognize an opportunity to set new goals for yourself, to look to the future, to give yourself permission to seek pleasure, to form new relationships, and generally enjoy life again. As we said earlier, doing this is no betrayal of the relationship you once enjoyed with the person you have lost. You need to accept that if you do establish new goals and new relationships, they can be enriched by the learning you gained from your previous experiences.

# 10
## Communicating and Comforting

With cancer, as in other areas of life, real and effective communication is very important. 'Real Communication' is not some kind of trendy jargon – it is about ordinary things like talking, listening, hearing, understanding, touching, feeling, comforting, honesty, and sensitivity.

Most people communicate effectively without even realizing they are doing so. It means responding naturally, and it is this natural response that people often forget is the most important part of caring for someone who is ill. This chapter highlights the importance of being aware of these natural skills, and making sure that they don't get swamped by anxiety. Such skills are intuitive, but must be encouraged if they are to flourish.

### *Physical contact*

When caring for young children with cancer, physical contact is very often the only means of communicating warmth, comfort, and concern. Children who are upset respond immediately to the hug, to the protection of a warm body. Take the opportunities presented during the day to hold a child close, to read a story, or envelop them after bathtime. These communications are very powerful, and ensure that the child remains secure inside and emotionally connected to others.

Children in hospital are often physically separated from loved ones by the necessary accompaniments of treatment, tubes, drips, etc. Hugging and cuddling may be impeded, but stroking, hand-holding, and light massaging of limbs are all important means of communication that need to occur at every available opportunity. Older children will need this too, even though they may have gone past the age when they would invite it if they were fit. Children under stress very often regress to an earlier stage of development; they feel very frightened and vulnerable, and need to be reassured by those actions that gave them comfort when they were younger.

Children often miss out on the day-to-day physical closeness that should be theirs as of right in families where attention is directed to another family member who is ill. However, children's needs cannot be shelved during a period of crisis. In fact, if the adults in the family are feeling under pressure, then the children are likely to feel the pressure even more – because they will not have the information and understanding that is available to the adults. They won't necessarily have the words to convey that they hurt inside, and are frightened that it may be their turn next to be seriously ill. They may be separated from one or other parent for the first time, and as far as they are concerned it may be a permanent separation. Temporary arrangements for care that may seem quite appropriate to an adult can seem like a life sentence or a punishment to a child, who feels abandoned. The period of crisis makes extra comfort and reassurance extremely necessary – it is a time when someone must take responsibility for devoting most of their time and energy to the healthy, but frightened, children in the family. Adults also regress when they are involved in a crisis, and need the same kind of comfort that is so important to a child.

The most basic way of comforting anyone in distress of any kind is physical contact. Physical contact is immediate and potent. It symbolizes the care of one person for another; it at once brings a feeling of comfort – and takes away the magnitude of the stress or anxiety that the distressed person may be feeling. Just the very act of taking someone in your arms and holding them may be sufficient to enable them to let go of strong pent-up feelings. Neither the person who releases the feelings, nor the person who triggers the release, should be at all embarrassed if this occurs. Just let it happen, and allow the expression of feeling to take its course without interruption, and without you necessarily feeling the need to offer verbal reassurance.

## The need to talk;
## the value of listening

Often, when a person has been able to let go in this way, they will be able to talk about many of the things that trouble them, and they should be allowed to do this. At this moment, the person just wants to talk and needs someone to listen. The person listening has no obligation to say or do anything to try to make things better; just allow the expression of feeling and the talking to flow. If a person says they feel utterly depressed, that life is not worth living, that they feel completely unworthy, or that they are frightened that they will die, don't argue with them. They just need to be allowed to put their thoughts and feelings into words. They are going through a process of sorting out a whole jumble of things that have caused confusion and upset inside. Eventually, they will sort out this jumble and upset for themselves. Anything you say will probably make no difference whatsoever at this stage. They are talking and you are listening, and interruptions to refute what they are saying – or to deny that they have any reason to feel as they do – can only block these very valuable outpourings. The outpourings are valuable to the distressed person. They may be painful for the listener, who would rather not hear some of the things being said, but the distressed person must be allowed to say them without interruption.

## Mutual comfort

You may feel helpless from time to time about your ability to bring comfort in times of pain or distress, and stand by feeling frustrated, thinking 'What can I do to help?' It may distress you to see someone crying because of some emotional turmoil, and instinctively your embarrassment may prompt you to urge them to stop crying, and not let things upset them. If you are embarrassed about the crying, then it doesn't help to make the distressed person feel they are causing you embarrassment. It may have taken a long time to get to this point of release, especially if crying has never come easily to them.

Being close physically helps to relieve the stress of both people in the partnership, and brings a feeling of calmness and wholeness. To the person who is ill, this warmth of physical comfort is very reassuring, and does much to repair damaged self-esteem and feelings of unworthiness.

Anyone who is ill or distressed can find comfort from the physical closeness of sharing a bed with their partner. There may be times when this is not possible for practical reasons, and there may be periods when physical contact cannot be tolerated, but these will be few and far between. From time to time, partners may think it best to move out of the marital bed – for instance, if the sick person has disturbed nights and both are suffering from sleeplessness and fatigue. In this case, every opportunity should be taken to enjoy physical closeness during the day.

It helps too, when you are lying together, to place your warm hands on your partner. Trust your own intuition, and put your hands wherever you feel they will help your partner most, or ask them to indicate where they would like you to hold them. Hands placed on the small of the back, the chest, or the stomach can encourage relaxation, and help to slow down and deepen the breathing – with the result that tension can be eased. While in this position, begin to tune into your partner's breathing, and then slow down your own breathing and begin to breathe more deeply. Eventually, your partner will respond by matching your breathing pattern. This can be very calming for both of you, and induce sleep in a restless person.

If the person in distress knows about diaphragmatic breathing, now is the time to remind them of it. If not, don't worry – just suggest breathing out as much as possible, breathing in again, and then encouraging the person to expel the air forcibly from the lungs. This is most effective for anyone feeling tense or in pain.

Similar calming and comforting techniques can be used even if you are not on such intimate terms with each other. It is very easy to hold the wrist, or the wrist with one hand and the back of the neck with the other, putting your fingers on the pulses at the front of the wrist and then, as you talk quietly, breathe more deeply.

Gradually, slow down and deepen your own breathing. It helps during this time not only to talk quietly and calmly, but gradually to slow down your rate of speaking. You can of course carry out the breathing technique without talking. This is very comforting to anyone at any time, but even more so to someone in pain or who may be agitated.

Gentle massage is another effective way of easing stress, and it is to be advocated not only for those who are ill, but for those caring for them. Gently massaging the feet, or even just holding them, can have a sedative effect, and softly stroking around the eyes, forehead, and cheeks can be very soothing. Stroking down the length of the arms and hands while holding your partner's hand in your other hand encourages relaxation. You can use the thumb of your holding hand to massage gently the back of your partner's hand. Similarly, you can stroke the legs and feet. Try using perfumed body oils with your massage; the aromas that are breathed in are pleasurable and aid relaxation. It is suggested that the massage is kept gentle, and away from those parts of the body obviously affected by the cancer, or which are very tender to the touch.

If you are the patient, and are living alone or there is no one available at home to offer you massage, then you might find it useful to treat yourself to a professional massage or an aromatherapy session. Foot massage or a visit to a professional reflexologist can be most soothing, and promotes the all-important 'feel-good factor'.

At this point, I want to put in a reminder that we are not talking solely of benefits to the patient. It is just as important, for their well-being, that the carers receive similar comforting and stress-relieving treatment from someone close to them. Someone in the family must take responsibility for caring for the principal carers. At best, carers must survive the process of caring without their own physical and mental resources being overstretched. It is no use driving yourself to complete the course of caring, and then having an emotional or physical breakdown.

## Pacing your day

It helps to arrange for all members of the family to have daily quiet times together – perhaps listening to favourite music or even a story cassette. If visitors arrive, invite them to join you. Tell them that is a quiet time and that it is essential that it remains so. You don't have to wear yourself out making cups of tea or regaling them with the story of the illness and its treatment – or even searching for 'safe' areas of conversation.

## The importance of talking about feelings

Strong emotions produce physical sensations, creating discomfort, tension, and even pain. One of the most disabling emotions anyone can have is anger, and if you are facing the crisis of life-threatening illness, then you have a lot to be angry about! It has stopped the normal progression of your life in its tracks, and you are bound to feel wretched inside. You may not even recognize that these uncomfortable feelings are a result of anger; but if you do not recognize it as such, then you will not be able to express it straightforwardly or talk about it. It may be that you explode at unsuspecting members of the family over something trivial. You may be constantly on edge, taking everything too seriously, fighting back tears, unable to laugh, or retreating into silence. If someone offends you, you may find you are unable to tell them directly, but instead fume inside, feeling resentment and hatred for the offender. Your anger and your attempts to suppress it may be creating a barrier between you and those who may be in a position to offer help. Anger, like anxiety and fear, is energy-consuming and disabling, and can turn inwards to eat away at your strength. Suppressed anger is destructive and, above all else, it depresses the spirit. So recognize your anger – make a list of all the things you have lost as a result of the illness, and honestly face up to how you feel about the loss; and then ask yourself whether these previously unacknowledged feelings are contributing to your internal discomfort.

Other people may recognize that you are angry, but do not know how to help you. Every day they may be on the receiving end of your anger, but they may not be the real cause of it. We all know about the difficult patient whose drink may be too hot, or too cold, who has too many blankets, or too few; who may protest long and loud if a request to a busy carer is not responded to immediately. Their anger may not necessarily be related to these things, but to the position they find themselves in. Most of us have had this experience when we've been in bed for a few days with flu – just think how much more deeply seated the anger must be if someone feels they may not get out of bed ever again.

There are occasions, though, when carers must indicate that certain behaviour is not acceptable and that good manners must prevail. Rather than indulge in bouts of peevish retaliation, it is time to sit down and face up to what is really causing the anger. A quiet display of authority may be sufficient to enable the patient to recognize the cause of their feelings, and to begin to talk about those things that really concern them.

It may be that one of the reasons why we do not communicate our feelings or worries directly and openly is that we are afraid how these feelings may be received. We are afraid of looking foolish, or appearing weak. This fear of looking foolish or being silly often comes from our early childhood, when attempts to convey worries openly may have been rebuffed by our parents telling us not to be silly. We soon learn to bottle up our true feelings, and begin to express them through our behaviour. At a time of serious illness, it is important for someone in the family to recognize that it is time for the games to stop. They cause confusion, and waste a lot of energy that is needed to cope with healing and caring.

Everyone must recognize the importance of direct communication, and to ensure that all members of the family are able to say honestly what is concerning them. They need to feel they are in a safe environment, and be assured that nothing they say will be considered silly or unimportant, or that others will be defensive if they feel they are being criticized.

## Real listening

Have you noticed how often people begin to respond to someone else's comment before the first person has even finished speaking? When this happens, it is a sure indication that the 'listener' is not really listening. Real communication is about listening fully to everything that is being said to you, then pausing long enough to take it all in, and then formulating a reply that acknowledges the content and spirit of what is being said.

As an exercise, next time you are in a group of people, just become an observer for a time and listen to the interplay that goes on between the members of the group. You will find that people are constantly responding to part communications. No wonder there are so many misunderstandings. We need to listen *fully* to everything that is being said without taking up a stance before the communication has been completed. It is important for people to learn how to do this whatever is happening in their lives, but it is even more important when people are facing the stress and uncertainty of cancer.

If you feel locked into a situation where no one really listens to each other, and if you feel that your chances of changing this for the benefit of everyone concerned are minimal, then look for help outside the family. Effective listeners can be found in support groups, among the clergy, among professional social workers, and, hopefully, your doctor. Others who have been through the whole process as patients or carers can also be extremely effective listeners, because they have experienced at first hand the dynamics of the family under stress. Another reason for seeking outside help is that sometimes your chosen confidante can help you to find ways of opening up more effective channels of communication within the family group. Listening to only part-communications, or communicating through a range of behaviours that demand that everyone else indulges in this unsatisfactory process of mind-reading, benefits no one. It is much better for someone to take the risk, and to insist on open, direct communication.

Have you ever noticed in a family how things can go from bad to worse, for days or even weeks on end, and then suddenly a slight incident will trigger an explosion of emotion – in other words, a flaming row. However, this flaming row will often lead people to say honestly what has been bothering them for some time. Confidences will be shared and, once the air has been cleared, communication between family members, for a time at least, will be easier. If this is the only way to get some honesty into the situation, so be it. This is a drastic way to relieve tension, though, and there is always the danger that someone will get hurt – so try to achieve better communication before things get to this point.

# 11

## Coping with Pain,
## Fear, and Anxiety

### *Understanding pain*

If you or a member of your family have cancer, I have no doubt that
high on your list of worries is the inevitability that pain must
accompany the illness. It is important, therefore, to have some
understanding of the nature of pain and the way it is relieved.

The main purpose of this chapter is to reassure you that it is not
necessary to suffer continuous, unrelieved severe pain at any stage
of the illness. Cancer pain can be treated, and there is no reason why
anyone undergoing treatment for the disease should have excessive
pain. If they have, then the doctor should be informed immediately.
The aim of pain control in cancer is to anticipate it, and to ensure
that it is kept in check at all times. What is important is that there is
freedom from pain to allow a good night's sleep. Disturbed sleep
results in exhaustion, and exhaustion limits a person's ability to fight
the illness; and is often the beginning of a vicious circle that involves
pain, disturbed sleep, more pain, etc.

Pain control is also concerned with providing complete relief
whether you are at rest during the day, walking, or moving around
generally. It is important that activity should be maintained as long
as possible, and that pain does not interfere with your appetite and
ability to enjoy a good quality of life. Even though you may have a
serious illness, absence from pain may mean that you can continue
to enjoy hobbies, outings, country walks, shopping visits, and all
those other things that add up to a rich life. There is no reason why
you should not continue driving unless your doctor recommends
otherwise. Freedom from pain is bound to reduce anxiety, and as
the anxiety is decreased, then your mood is likely to be more
cheerful, calm, and relaxed. This change of attitude will in turn help
to relieve any depression in you and in other members of the family.

Activity and rest may need to be balanced very carefully to avoid
getting over-tired or stressed. Sometimes pain will increase when
people overdo things, so it is important to be sensible about the
amount of activity undertaken. It is probably better to do this than

103

to increase the amount of medication you take, which will further reduce your capacity to move about and think clearly. Even if you have been told by your doctors that your cancer is terminal, then it is still realistic to expect a pain-free end.

### Cancer does not automatically cause pain

In fact, many cancers, even at an advanced stage, do not cause pain; and one of the problems about cancer is that it can reach an advanced stage without the pain signal alerting us. It is very often other symptoms that tell us that something needs attention. This is quite different from most other injuries or illness, where pain or discomfort is nearly always the warning sign that something is wrong. Therefore pain is normally a late symptom of cancer, arising usually when secondary cancers or metastases spread to other parts of the body, particularly into the bones. Sometimes it is the spinal column that is attacked, and the resulting collapse of the bones in this area can cause nerves to be trapped. Pain often results when a cancer grows and causes obstruction to one of the organs of the body. However, you have to bear in mind that in spite of this, only two-thirds of people with widespread cancer have any pain.

There may be pain arising from necessary forms of treatment; for example, following surgery there may be residual pain from adhesions, scar tissue, or damage to nerves. Radiotherapy may produce slight damage to tissue in the area of radiation, and pain can result. Help will be necessary while this lasts. Chemotherapy may also be responsible for some pain. Most forms of treatment can give rise to some pain and discomfort, which ranges from moderate to acute. Some pain may continue for a long time after healing has taken place, producing a chronic pain state. This may need quite different treatment from other kinds of pain. You will probably find that if you can do some exercise and learn effective relaxation techniques, you will find it easier to cope with chronic pain. (For a full discussion of these forms of treatment, you may find it helpful to read my book *Coping Successfully with Pain*, Sheldon Press, 1992.)

Individual responses to pain vary greatly, and most of us are psychologically keyed up to anticipate a greater amount of pain than is actually experienced. Although pain is a physical sensation, the amount of pain you feel depends very much on the situation in which you experience it. You can even choose to ignore it, consciously or unconsciously.

From experience, you probably know that if you have been

playing sport and have received a knock, you have quite happily carried on playing, disregarding the discomfort you are feeling. At that time, the game was more important than the pain. You may also have noticed that you can carry on certain activities with a reasonable amount of comfort, while at other times the pain increases. Many men can happily enjoy a day's fishing, but find their pain excruciating if they have to visit shops! Women may find shopping for food brings on pain, whereas buying a new outfit may be quite pleasurable. I normally have difficulty sitting or standing for more than a few minutes at a time, and these activities cause me great distress and discomfort. However, I have noticed that when I have an easel and paintbrush in front of me, I get so involved, and time goes so quickly, that I am completely unaware of any discomfort. When I am painting, I can stand or sit for a couple of hours quite happily. Sometimes I do feel a lot of discomfort at the end of a painting session, but the enjoyment that I have had stays with me for such a long time that I feel as though I have earned the pain!

Inactivity, boredom, and negative feelings generally lead to a greater perception of pain. It has been found that in these situations the production of endorphins, the body's own natural pain-killers, is reduced, thereby limiting a person's capacity to cope with pain. A lot depends on how you feel about your pain, and it is quite common for people to talk about 'suffering' from pain. Suffering relates not only to the pain sensation itself, but to your feelings, thoughts, and behaviour resulting from the pain. Because there is a very close relationship between the mind and the body, these subjective elements can be responsible for prolonging your pain, and possibly even increasing it.

The mind plays a very important part, because we have the capacity to imagine and anticipate the future. Anticipation and imagination can prompt us to think, 'If the pain is bad now, and I am losing the ability to do the things I enjoy, what is it going to be like in the next few weeks, months, or even years?' This will prompt anxiety and tension, which will then exacerbate the pain. Talking about pain and dwelling on it will also reinforce the pain sensation. As you talk about your pain and remember times when things have been difficult, you trigger off memories that can actually bring about physiological changes that make the pain real.

How we think about pain has a great deal of influence on our ability to deal with it. If we know that pain normally accompanies certain injuries or illnesses, and is likely to recede as we get better, then most of us have no difficulty accepting the fact of the pain and taking it in our stride, with or without the help of a few pain-killers. We don't worry about it too much, or think it will cause a major upset in our lives. I'm sure that if you have ever broken an arm or wrist or sprained an ankle, you probably made a fuss about it for a day or so, but you had an expectation that in due course things would get better and the pain would subside. With proper medical treatment, the pain diminished, you accepted the limitations of the injury, and resumed normal activities as quickly as possible.

Some illnesses such as cancer already involve a great deal of negative thought, so when pain arises there is a tendency to develop negative thoughts about your ability to cope with the pain. Fear and pessimistic expectations about the future challenge people's belief in their ability to cope with all that is involved in the illness. You may even feel that the onset of pain is a signal for you to surrender to the pain and the illness, and just throw in the towel. You may assume you will not be able to deal with the pain, that it will always be present, and that it is likely to get worse. The fear is added to as you and your family *mistakenly* equate the severity of the pain with the increasing seriousness of the illness. When such thoughts are entertained, the pain is felt more intensely, leading to fear and feelings of helplessness.

With an increase in helplessness you can feel as though nothing that you can do can influence your pain. You have lost control. At this point, there may be demands for larger and stronger doses of medication. But when there is such a strong emotional element to pain, it is quite likely that the medication at this stage will not do the job effectively. You may feel even more helpless, believing that no one or nothing can help – and, because of the strong medication, be unable to participate in those activities that can bring so much benefit psychologically and socially. Helplessness and feelings of despair add to the perception of pain, and increase tension and fear, and consequently the intensity and duration of the pain. This pain/fear cycle needs to be recognized and broken. The medical professionals need to be in touch with the influence of these strong psychological elements in order to advise or call in appropriate outside support.

Fear is not always acknowledged directly, for some people suppress fear about the illness. They may not even admit it to themselves, and in so doing lay the foundations of depression and further pain. Some may actually admit the fear to themselves, but hide it from their family, not wanting to burden them. The barriers between the family members and the patient then grow, and those who are in the best position to help can't break them down. The family may feel inadequate to offer help – but they can, just by indicating they are ready to listen if the patient feels the need to talk. The emphasis must always be on reducing fear and easing anxiety and tension.

## *Easing the fear*

One of the greatest services that any human being can do for another is to take away their fear. When I teach people how this can be done there is usually surprise and wonder at the simplicity of it. There is no need for sophisticated medical or psychological techniques. Each one of us has the capacity to take away another person's fear; and each one of us has the capacity to take away our own fear.

We need to talk calmly and in a relaxed way, our own calmness conveys itself to the one who hurts, and there is a recognition by the sufferer that there is someone there who understands their fear. The relief is immediate, and feelings of panic are taken away. This is a real 'first-aid treatment', and no one can take away its importance. The interesting thing is that it doesn't seem to matter what you say, so long as you talk quietly and calmly. There is something very soothing about the human voice, and it is this quality that is latched on to by someone who is in distress. It helps as you are talking to divert attention from what is going on here and now by reminding the person in pain of a more pleasant time, a more pleasant experience, an event that has been shared. If you are very familiar with the person, you have no doubt shared happy moments, holidays together, or visited places that have a special meaning. This is the time when you might introduce the words, 'Do you remember when . . .?', and then go on to talk about some of these happier things. You might even try, once the initial fear is over, reading aloud to them or playing some of their favourite music. What is important is that you stay with them until the crisis is over. Such expressions of care and concern may be vital in preventing the vicious circle of pain – tension – fear – helplessness – pain. (You may want to re-read the previous chapter, which gives various suggestions for offering comfort to someone in distress.)

As carer, you may have difficulty in keeping your own panic and anxiety under control. It is not easy to do this if you are facing this kind of crisis for the first time. In fact, you may always have been a person who 'gets into a flap' in times of emergency. If you know this, then it is helpful to have someone else who is reliable and has a calming influence to call upon, maybe a neighbour or a friend on the end of the telephone, or even a Helpline. Knowing that someone is on hand or nearby is often enough to support you and give you the confidence to deal with the situation. It is important that you do not convey your alarm by your words or behaviour, as this can serve to add to the fears of the ill person. Remember that the techniques that I am advising as being helpful to use with other people will work equally well with yourself. You can follow your own internal script, reminding yourself about your breathing, telling yourself to slow down, and to reach out calmly, taking the hand or embracing the sufferer. Nothing more is expected from you – the important thing is that you are there. Many people surprise themselves during times of crisis at their ability to remain calm and provide help and support. Often, it is worse thinking about the prospect than it is when faced with the real situation. (The next chapters expand on some of these ideas, and explains how you can take control of your own emotions whether you are a patient or a carer.) The emphasis is on learning relaxation skills that play a fundamental part in the total treatment of someone with cancer by reducing anxiety and tension. As anxiety and tension diminish, feelings of pain can also be reduced. Learning to reduce fear is equally important for patient and carer.

Once the fear and anxiety have been controlled, it is possible to develop other ways of managing pain. People who concentrate on their pain and are constantly on the alert, waiting for the onset of painful sensations, do become more aware of their pain. It is possible to divert attention from painful sensations. In other words, to fill the mind with so many interesting things that there is no room left for the pain. Pain, therefore, is a problem particularly for people who are under-stimulated, who have little to do, and use their time and energy in paying attention to painful sensations.

Maintaining involvement in pleasurable activities and hobbies is important. It is unfortunate that in the crisis of diagnosis and the early days of the illness, people retreat into isolation – and at this point abandon work, hobbies, social activities, and many of the things that keep us absorbed and free from worry. Often we don't do this through choice. We spend long periods waiting for hospital appointments, waiting for results of tests, recovering from spells in hospital, and the effects of treatment. It is almost as though we have been given a new career, but it is not a career that brings rewards – it has with it long spells of inactivity, boredom, and time for anxiety and fear to take root as we reflect on those things that we have lost, and the horrors that might be ahead of us. This is a time when pain can creep up on us, and the vicious circle of pain, tension, fear, pain, takes hold once again. It is a time, too, when, because of enforced inactivity, the body begins to lose tone, muscles waste, and general fitness diminishes. This has nothing at all to do with the effects of the illness, but is a result of inactivity. When the body is in this low state, it is easy for pain to become established. With movement, muscles unaccustomed to use become sore and stiff, we become breathless and easily fatigued, leading to the desire to rest and do less. You can easily see from this how we can build up another vicious circle.

## Mind and body versus pain

What is needed at this stage is to gradually get back into regular physically and mentally absorbing activity – and this is where the family can help enormously. The patient's mind must be kept stimulated, and the body must be reconditioned. It is possible to work towards this fitness of mind and body at most stages of the illness, perhaps pausing only when the worst effects of treatment are present. The healthier our mental and physical state, the more able we are to combat the effects of the illness and infections, and stay free from pain. One of the problems faced by a sick person is that of over-protection. For many of us, 'being ill' equates with being inactive, being looked after, staying indoors, having someone to cook our meals, and to fetch and carry. The key is finding the correct balance between rest and activity.

It is important to seek out those people who offer stimulation. We have all been grateful sometime, when we have been low, for the services of a friend who has the innate ability to take us out of ourselves. We all know someone who just has to appear and our spirits lift. Their conversation stimulates us to feel better, and when they go, we feel as though we have had a holiday. We definitely need a lot of friends like this! Just think of what an uplift it gives us when we anticipate a surprise outing? Getting washed and dressed in smart clothes, going out into normal company –

perhaps even taking responsibility for paying the bill. Being absorbed in this way gives a tremendous boost to the spirit.

These various techniques of managing pain may be sufficient for most people for much of the time, but for some it may be necessary to be helped by medication. The pain management methods just described can be used quite safely in conjunction with medication, and they may even help to limit the amount of medication needed.

## *Monitoring your pain*

It is important to be as precise as possible when describing pain to those managing your illness, for this will enable them to give the appropriate help. From my own experience, and from working with people with pain, I know how difficult it is to describe the kind of pain you have and to pinpoint the source of it. It is very helpful if you can make a note when you experience pain, perhaps just by jotting down odd words that describe what the pain feels like – for instance, a pressure, a stabbing, a tightness, a cramp? These are important indications to your doctor as to the cause of the pain. It is useful to indicate whether the pain comes in waves, the intervals between the waves, whether the pain comes following certain activities such as bending or walking, and how long it lasts. It may be that the pain comes either just before or just after eating. All these points are important. It is also useful to keep a diary of your pain. Many people think they have constant pain, but when they begin to monitor their pain they find that the level is always changing.

It is most important to note:

- at what time of day your pain is at its highest level;
- at what time of day your pain is at its lowest level.

It is also important to note the following:

- Has something happened to upset you?
- Have you missed a meal?
- Have you had visitors who have perhaps over-extended their stay?
- Have you missed an afternoon rest?
- Have you spent a day lounging around watching television for many hours, and missed out on some physical activity and exercise?

- Have you waited until the pain has taken hold before taking your medication?

## *Medication*

For severe cancer pain, morphine and its derivatives are the most widely used drugs. They are simple to administer, and provide good pain relief for most people.

Morphine acts directly on a centre in the brain and spinal cord in order to interrupt the pain signal. However, some pain is more localized and needs an additional form of medication, such as aspirin or paracetamol, to work in conjunction with the morphine. Some people are also troubled by muscle spasms, and in these cases muscle relaxants may also be given in addition to morphine.

In most cases, though, cancer pain is not a major problem, and only a mild pain-killer may be needed. People with cancer can suffer in the same way as people without it do: aching muscles, headaches, or other problems that cause mild pain. However, when you have cancer, these pains can often cause anxiety, and it may be that –along with the mild pain-killer – reassurance is needed. Therefore, do not hesitate to report these pains to your doctor should they arise.

You and your family may become very upset if morphine is prescribed. Somehow we tend to associate being on morphine with having a limited number of days to live, for it has a bad image from the past. However, you need not be so pessimistic. Morphine is usually prescribed when aspirin and codeine, used by themselves, are no longer sufficient to control the pain. The amount of time that morphine may be needed will vary from individual to individual. Some may need it for only a matter of days, others for weeks, months, or even years. The amount of time is not important, so long as the person remains comfortable and able to live life as fully as possible. There is no evidence that morphine, used as prescribed, hastens death – but there is plenty of evidence that it can increase a person's quality of life.

You may get worried about taking strong pain-killing drugs on a regular basis, but there is no need to worry that these will be addictive. If strong pain-killing drugs are prescribed for cancer, then you can be sure that they are needed. However, if morphine is stopped suddenly, then there will be problems; when it is no longer needed for pain control, your doctor will advise on how to reduce the dosage gradually.

The biggest danger in taking morphine is that of adopting a 'macho' approach – that is, seeing how much pain you can bear before taking the next dose. This is not at all sensible. Experience shows that sticking to a regular timetable, usually every four hours, provides the best combination of good pain relief with least side-effects. If you take it only when you feel you need it, you will suffer alternating periods of comfort and pain. This is no way to achieve and maintain a good quality of life. If you delay taking your medication until the pain returns, you will have to wait 30–40 minutes before the medication begins to take effect and the pain eases. You end up making your own and everybody else's life a misery, and this is avoidable, unnecessary pain.

If the regular dosage prescribed is not sufficient to ease your pain, are you pacing yourself properly? Are you tackling too much before you take a break? Are you living under emotional strain? Be honest with yourself, and think about any changes you might make in the way you structure your day. Talk over your worries with someone. It may also be necessary to discuss with your doctor the possibility of reducing the interval between doses; this is particularly important for controlling the pain at night. It is usually recommended that you have an increased dose before settling down to sleep, take a further dose on waking, and then resume your previous timetable. For example, if your timetable decrees that you have a dose at 8.00 p.m., and you wish to turn out the light at 10.00 p.m., then take another dose then. On waking, say at 6.00 a.m., take another dose, and then if your normal doseage time is 8.00 a.m., resume at that time – do not wait until 10.00 a.m. If you have *any* problems concerning your medication, then you *must* discuss them with your your district nurse, Macmillan nurse, or doctor.

People get very confused about their medication, particularly if there are many different prescription drugs involved with various aspects of their treatment, or maybe they are taking medication for a quite separate medical condition – for example, high blood pressure or diabetes. Do not make any decisions about which drugs to take and which not to take without having a full discussion with your medical adviser about the importance of every item of medication that has been prescribed. Once you start making independent and uninformed decisions about which medication *you* think you ought or ought not to take, you may be cutting off the major source of your pain control. Sometimes there may be pain, and the doctor may be getting blamed for it – but it may be that you are not carrying out his instructions in taking the correct medicine at the proper intervals.

All drugs that bring relief from pain have some side-effects, but these can usually be treated. The most common side-effect is constipation, and it is probably best to ask your doctor to prescribe the necessary laxatives and stool softeners along with your medication. Changes in diet can also help you – make sure that there is plenty of fibre in your diet and that you eat things like tinned peaches in syrup, cooked dried prunes, and dried apricots. Fruit taken in this way is less acidic than fresh fruit, and you may be able to tolerate it more easily. You may also be advised to counter the dehydrating effects of certain drugs by taking in more liquid. This can also help considerably in easing the discomfort of constipation. If you do get problems from constipation, always mention it to your doctor, district nurse, or Macmillan nurse – whoever you are most in contact with. They are quite accustomed to dealing with such problems, and will be able to give you something that offers speedy relief.

Part of your pain treatment may involve reducing the size of the cancerous mass that is putting pressure on organs, and therefore causing pain. It may be suggested to you that you have some radiotherapy or chemotherapy in order to achieve this.

## Managing your pain

Every hospital district is served by a Pain Clinic, and it may be that you will be referred to such a clinic if the cancer has affected the nerves in any part of your body. Pressure on nerves can cause persistent, long-lasting pain, which may continue long after your body has healed. It is possible to administer injections or oral drugs that 'block off' the nerves that are affected.

It may be that your pain can be controlled without the use of drugs, or with help additional to the use of drugs. In recent years, a great deal of relief has been brought to people by the use of the TENS machine (Transcutaneous Electronic Nerve Stimulation). This consists of a small unit, about the size of a telephone pager, which is connected by two or more fine wires to rubber electrodes positioned on or near the site of the pain. The unit is powered by a small battery, and electrical impulses have the effect of cutting out the pain signal before it reaches the brain. TENS is quite safe to use, and produces no harmful side-effects. I have been using one for spinal pain for almost ten years now, and would gladly recommend anyone with persistent pain to consider this form of pain relief.

Pain is often a subject addressed by some of the many support groups that have been set up to help cancer patients and their families. It is possible through such groups to learn effective pain management skills, particularly that of relaxation. There is a growing move to extend to other areas of the country the pioneering pain management course established at Walton Hospital in Liverpool some twelve years ago. The concentration there is on encouraging patients with long-term pain to develop as many approaches to managing their pain as possible. You will need to keep in touch with your own doctor to find out more about centres such as this in your area.

# 12

## Recognizing Stress

The diagnosis and experience of cancer and its treatment bring dramatic changes. Behaviour and habits established over the years are completely overturned; ambitions and aspirations have to be reviewed – not just for the person with the illness, but for everyone closely involved. Everybody's energy is directed towards the cancer. Sometimes the stress of the change can be so strong that family members 'take flight'; they are unable to face the upheaval of it all, and focus their attention outside the family. Yet however people react, there is no escaping the fact that change is unavoidable – and change often means stress.

In the case of serious illness such as cancer, family members and patients experience many situations that are stressful in themselves. You will understand this much more easily if I list just a few of the things that can cause stress: hospital visits for out-patient appointments; the ordeal of medical tests; the waiting for results; the anticipation of the diagnosis; the confirmation of the diagnosis; the fear of treatment procedures; visits to the hospital for treatment; side-effects of treatment and drugs; changes in physical appearance as a result of surgery or chemotherapy; lack of sensitivity encountered in professionals, family members, and friends; fatigue caused by doing too much or resulting from disturbed nights, fear of the recurrence of cancer, or confirmation of reccurrence; keeping secrets; and being overwhelmed by endless conflicting advice from well-meaning friends and relatives. Stress can also arise from feeling helpless and out of control – feeling that the management of your life is completely in the hands of the professionals, and that the course of the illness is itself uncertain.

At this point, even those of us who have lived positively and have learned many effective ways of coping with problems in the past can feel the full impact of our impotence. Realistically, it may seem that we have only a limited number of options available, feeling that our capacity to enjoy many experiences has been taken away. In addition to the illness itself, there may be limitations imposed by it: being unable to work, to get out of the house, to drive, walk, or do much for ourselves. As a result of these things, it is easy to suffer from lack of stimulation. This can bring about feelings of depression

115

and stress. At this time, it is very difficult to see how the skills learned during a lifetime of coping can help us now with the frustration, fear, and loss.

## How do we recognize stress in ourselves or others?

I have already mentioned some of the things to look out for. Fear and anxiety are to a certain extent an unavoidable part of any life-threatening illness and its treatment. They are emotions shared by everyone involved, and such feelings can result in excessive fatigue, muscular aches and pains, headaches, digestive upsets, shallow breathing, disturbed sleep, and a range of other physical and emotional disorders.

Stress also alters our ability to tolerate frustration, to think clearly, and it interferes with our perception of what is going on around us. Innocent remarks may be interpreted as hostile, or as challenges to our competence. The result may be that someone of normally calm temperament flies off the handle, or dissolves into uncharacteristic floods of tears.

Do not feel overwhelmed by this catalogue of the many potential stresses which accompany cancer. They do not appear all at once and you will approach each situation as it arises – just as you have done through your life. Nor will everyone experience all of these things as stressful, but it is understandable that from time to time things will get on top of you, whether you are the patient or a member of the family. It is important to remember that life goes on and good experiences will continue to happen to every member of the family during the course of the illness. New friendships will be established, new places visited, new hobbies tried.

We have already seen from examples in the book how Arthur responded to the exceptional burdens put upon him by uncharacteristic excessive drinking. Anna found comfort in 'bingeing' on chocolate, while Peggy sought help via medication.

The story of Peter and Lillian will illustrate that reactions to stress may not always immediately be recognized as such.

## Peter and Lillian's story

When she was in her middle 20s, Lillian developed skin cancer. She was assured that it was not life-threatening and after a short course of treatment the problem cleared up, except for a discoloured patch on her neck. To onlookers it was hardly noticeable, however Lillian seemed to lose all confidence in herself, and developed an aversion to her own image. She found it difficult to look at herself in the mirror and hid the offending blemish with high-necked jumpers, summer and winter. She gave up all social activity outside the home. Until the time of her illness, Lillian had played a major part in joining Peter in social activities connected with his job. They were often invited to company functions where it seemed important that a wife was fully supportive of her husband's career. When Lillian returned to work, she had periods of feeling sick which meant that she had to come home. After persevering for three months she gave up work altogether and remained firmly indoors. Meanwhile, her husband Peter worried about the change that had come over Lillian and, concerned that the situation was getting out of hand, sought professional help, and for some months Lillian received treatment from a clinical psychologist. Very gradually the situation eased and Lillian developed more confidence, was able to resume work, and enjoyed going out again.

This seemed to be the end of the story until two years later Peter developed a severe rash on the back of his hands and arms and on his feet. For some time he was treated with creams and lotions to no avail. His GP then referred Peter to a consultant dermatologist whose investigations suggested the problem may be emotional rather than physical. Peter then underwent a course of psychological treatment in order to pin-point the cause. For the first time since his wife became ill, Peter was able to talk openly about his fears and anxieties for his wife and for their future together. He had found it easier to cope with the physical illness of his wife by concentrating on practical issues like doing all the shopping and cooking, paying the bills, driving his wife for her treatment sessions. What he had found difficult was the emotional response of his wife to her illness and her feeling about herself afterwards. It was a time of great frustration and helplessness. He felt that there was nothing he could do which would convince her that neither he nor anyone else noticed any change in her appearance. His rational approach did nothing to deal with her emotional problem. He felt very embarrassed with colleagues at work who were aware of her illness and her successful treatment. They kept pressing him about bringing her along to the company dinners and he felt her absence was being interpreted as a sign of a rift in the marriage. Lillian did not suddenly get better, and Peter had a major task in supporting his wife through periods of doubt and failing confidence during the progress of her psychological treatment. Once it appeared that all anxieties had been put behind them, and it was time to relax and enjoy life once more, Peter's problem started. He was fortunate that his GP and the dermatologist were alert to the possibility that the problem had something to do with the emotional burden he had been carrying for some time and that it would respond to psychological treatment.

If you recognize that you or anyone in your family is showing signs of stress, then it is time to do something about it. Talking about the source of the stress and discomfort is important, but doing something about it is even more important. You may not be able to get rid of the cancer, but you can reduce your stress – whether you are patient or carer. In the following chapter we will look at something called 'deep relaxation', and how we can use it to reduce our stress levels.

# 13
## Keeping Going –
## Keeping Well

In the last chapter we looked at stress and its implications at all stages of the illness and during periods of remission. Everyone in this situation needs to accept that coping with illness is hard work. For this reason it is important for every member of the family, including the patient, to think about ways of maintaining their own general health. You have to think about the illness and its aftermath as being equivalent to a marathon race and pace yourself accordingly. It is important that you find ways to support the medical treatment by nurturing your own physical and emotional resources. Above all, it is important to recognize that you, as the patient – and your family – have an important part to play in your own treatment and survival. When you are in the middle of the crisis following the diagnosis and the early days of treatment it is very difficult to see what you can do in the process of healing.

I emphasize that this chapter is addressed to the family as a whole. You are all involved and have a responsibility to maintain your own health in order that you can care for each other.

I want to focus on three important, positive ways in which you can become active participants in the treatment and survival process:

- ensuring adequate nourishment
- exercise
- learning the skills of deep relaxation.

## *Ensuring adequate nourishment*

The onset of the illness and the ensuing treatment will bring about a need to think about the sort of diet which will help you maintain the best possible fitness during the treatment period and afterwards when you enter a period of recovery and remission. It will be helpful to consult your doctor and dietician and follow their recommendations. You and members of your family can find out as much as possible about diet by conducting your own research.

There will be periods when the appetite is depressed: following the shock of diagnosis, and at times when recovering from chemotherapy and radiotherapy treatment sessions. These can cause a great deal of anxiety to all family members. These are the times when you eat whatever you fancy. You will find that your medical advisers understand these problems and can provide a great deal of help with special foods which provide the necessary nutrition.

If you are caring for someone with cancer you have to be careful that your anxiety about the patient does not cause you to neglect your own nutritional needs. This can so easily happen at times of crisis. At the end of a two-month period of intensive caring I found that I had lost 28lbs in weight.

There is much debate at present about the importance of diet in the prevention of cancer and heart disease, and about the importance of thinking about the adoption of dietary changes during periods of remission in order to prevent a recurrence of cancer. It is very easy to become neurotic and over-fussy about your food; as a general rule it is important to include in your diet substantial portions of fruit and vegetables and cut back on saturated animal fats. Food and eating are basic to family life. What and when you eat is to a large extent dependent on family tastes and tradition, so the implications of any changes in diet will have to be considered by the family as a whole.

## Is there a case for exercise?

With illnesses like cancer, which can be prolonged and involve periods of quiescence interspersed with acute episodes, there is confusion about whether exercise should be done at all – and if so, how much. Traditionally, when someone is ill they are encouraged to rest and the family takes on a protective role, showing concern at the slightest effort the patient makes. This over-protective attitude, while understandable, is not always the most helpful.

There is increasing evidence to support the view that exercise is an important adjunct to treatment itself. The popular view about people with cancer is that they are weak and sick, but this is not inevitable. Patients who were given an exercise programme while on chemotherapy maintained and improved their fitness. Not only did they have an improved drainage of waste from their bodies but they tolerated their treatments with fewer side-effects. Follow-up studies indicate that patients involved in such programmes have a longer survival record. It is thought that an appropriate use of exercise helps to increase the energy needed to fight the cancer and the side-effects of chemotherapy. What is more, the immune system, depleted by chemotherapy, can be stimulated. In tests undertaken in the USA people involved in aerobic exercise programmes in conjunction with chemotherapy were shown to have an increased number of white blood cells throughout their treatment. White blood cells are, of course, the foundation of the immune system.

Exercise has also been shown to restore levels of white cells in those people whose blood count has dropped. When the blood cell count drops it is not possible to give patients the levels of chemotherapy needed to fight the illness. The exercises which are important during treatment are those which provide work for the heart and lungs: using an exercise bike, walking, swimming and, in some cases, jogging. People who were physically active before undergoing chemotherapy are encouraged to continue to enjoy these activities. The important thing for these people is that they learn to listen to their bodies and to assess for themselves when their energy is low. These low points follow immediately after chemotherapy treatments, so rest and relaxation for a few days before and after treatment is normally recommended.

There may be times when you do have to spend some time in bed as a necessary part of your treatment. There are a number of exercises which you can do at this time in order to maintain your strength and fitness. You can exercise toes and ankles, do arm and leg-raising exercises, sit-ups, shoulder shrugging, neck and head circling, as well as doing some breathing exercises. All these will help to speed up your recovery after treatment.

During periods of remission, many people find benefit from taking up some physical activity. The advantage of this is that most of the normal physical activities offer opportunities for social contact and as a result reduce isolation and depression. Dancing, yoga, swimming, walking, bowling, in fact anything which does not overtire you and provides you with opportunities, can be enjoyed. A friend of mine who had a mastectomy some 20 years ago resumed playing tennis regularly and still plays. This has not only strengthened her upper body muscles but has maintained a good level of fitness, improved her self-esteem, and has ensured pleasurable social contact.

Following operations, and at certain times during the illness, you will need to be guided by your doctor or physiotherapist who know when it is appropriate to move around and do some formal exercise. Exercise and activity contribute directly to the development of a positive approach. When you exercise, the brain produces chemicals (endorphins) which have the effect of making you feel better, as they relieve depression and increase the sense of well-being. A few minutes exercise can be effective in taking your mind off how bad you may be feeling. Irrespective of any physiological reaction, when you are sitting around brooding and anticipating the worst, you do not feel good. When you are active you feel better and your anxiety and stress are reduced.

Sometimes when you begin to move again after enforced rest, movement is painful and you may need some encouragement and help to control your fear. The worst thing you can do at this stage is to give up and decide to lead a completely restricted life. For most people this is frustrating and brings rage at the knowledge that physical disability is preventing you from enjoying even simple pleasures, so the message is DON'T GIVE UP!

## *What is deep relaxation?*

The practice of deep relaxation contributes directly to a reduction of stress, no matter what its cause. It is probably one of the most positive activities that can be undertaken together by all members of the family involved in coping with cancer.

You might imagine that deep relaxation is something that you do every time you sit down to watch the television, to read a newspaper, or to have a cigarette. This is not so – these merely offer a respite from normal working activity and are unlikely to relieve any feelings of distress and strong tensions within the body. In contrast, deep relaxation is a specific skill and, like all skills, you have to learn it and practise it regularly to build up its beneficial effects. We all knew how to relax as children, but most of us have forgotten how to do it. Fortunately, it can be re-learned.

Deep relaxation is a process during which you will allow all the tension to move away from every muscle and organ of your body, producing feelings of calmness and well-being. During deep relaxation the blood will flow more freely throughout your whole system. This improvement in circulation is beneficial to anyone who practises deep relaxation but, in particular, if you are having chemotherapy you will benefit in a number of specific ways:

- The drugs involved in treatment will be distributed around the body much more effectively.
- The body will be able to get rid of dead cancer cells much more quickly.
- Other waste products will be drained more efficiently, thus reducing any build-up of toxicity deriving from your medication.
- The lymph system will work more freely, and the result will be a more effective immune system so that the body's own ability to combat the disease will be strengthened.
- If you have pain, then the chemicals (endorphins) responsible for controlling it will be produced in greater abundance.

It is no use learning the skill of deep relaxation and using it only occasionally, for instance just before you are due to make a hospital visit. Of course, it is important to use it at this time, but its effectiveness will not be so great as when you make deep relaxation practice a daily and enjoyable feature of your life – something you look forward to, just as you look forward to a good meal or a warm bed. Although you may initially learn and practise your relaxation skills at home in a warm, quiet, darkened room, they can ultimately be used as and when you require them; for instance, you may use a relaxation tape in hospital while waiting for your appointment, or before, or during and after your chemotherapy session. Patients who regularly practise relaxation techniques say they experience less unpleasant side-effects of medication.

It is significant that people commonly talk about 'fighting' cancer. The very word 'fight' brings with it feelings of tension, aggression, and struggle. The word 'fight' may be appropriate when we think of the immune system attempting to destroy cancer cells, but the word is not useful when used to describe how we ourselves may assist in this process of healing. We are looking for a complete relaxation of tension. Relaxation, as the name suggests, brings respite from the 'fight' and enables us to recover the physical and emotional energy our bodies need to cope with illness and stress.

With relaxation you will begin to feel the confidence of having control over areas of your life that you thought had gone. Remember, you have nothing at all to lose from learning these skills and everything to gain. If you are in a position where you feel that options have been taken away because of a growing physical incapacity, then what better activity to follow than learning these new skills; they can only be beneficial.

An effective relaxation strategy enables those who practise it to develop positive thought-patterns which stop the flow of destructive, anxiety-provoking, tension-producing negative thought. It is important only to have those thoughts in your mind that you wish to be there! Learn to recognize when unwanted, troublesome thoughts stray into your mind. Don't let them take root. Let them go. Equip yourself with a repertoire of positive memories and pleasant thoughts to fill your mind.

A detailed programme of deep relaxation techniques can be found in my book *Coping Successfully with Pain*.

Of course, in real life things aren't as simple as just learning new techniques or making a few adjustments. There is little control over when things happen, and families are in a constant state of adjustment, re-evaluation, building and re-building, taking pleasure when they can and coping with difficulties as they arise. Learning new ways of living can take some time and there will be many set-backs.

## *Pat's story*

I first met Pat when she was 52. She had been referred by her GP because of a problem of residual pain following a mastectomy operation some eight years previously. He thought she might need to talk things through and to learn some effective relaxation techniques. The story is best told in Pat's own words.

'I remember the time well. My daughter Jean had been married to David for six months and we had just been out with them to celebrate the news that she was pregnant. My feeling is it was that night, when I was getting ready for bed, that I felt a lump in my breast, and it seemed as though in no time at all I had been through the investigations, had my breast removed, and was in the middle of a course of chemotherapy. I remember crying a lot, feeling very depressed, and quite ill at times. I think I even got to the stage where I was planning what would happen after my funeral. I found myself making lists for Bob, my husband, so that things would not be too difficult for him when he was left by himself. It was such a shock when I found I was doing this that I swore I would never get so low, and whenever I felt myself getting that way I would phone my daughter and we would talk for hours, planning for the time the baby would be born. This seemed to keep me going. My treatment went well and I was planning for a long convalescence before returning to my job as senior tracer in a drawing office. I was looking forward to helping my daughter with her new baby during this time. About a month before the baby was born, Bob walked in one night and said he had been made redundant and had only a month to work. It seemed then that all the anger that had been stored up in me while I had gone through my treatment burst out. I ranted and raved around the house, and even threw things. It upset Bob, I can tell you – he thought it was all aimed at him. He had never seen me like this before. I felt, after all I've been through, and now this coming on top of it; it was just like the DJ on the radio who says "When one door closes, another slams in your face!" When I had calmed down, Bob and I talked about how we would manage over the next 20 years before he could collect his retirement pension. We didn't know how much redundancy money he would get, and what savings we had had been eaten up during my illness and on our daughter's wedding. I could see nothing for it but for me to return to work as quickly as possible.

'Bob and Jean – and my doctor – tried to talk me out of it but I was determined. When I look at that decision in the cold light of day I realize what a foolhardy step it must have seemed. I hadn't worked for nearly a year, I had lost confidence about my appearance and about going out. I had not even got back to driving the car; I had very little strength down my right arm and side since the operation. Not very good for someone who spends seven hours a day at a drawing board! Before the month was up, I went back to work. My hair looked a mess, following the chemotherapy, and my clothes no longer fitted me properly. I was petrified at the prospect of meeting all my old colleagues. I hadn't even got my coat off before the boss called me into his office. "Pat," he said, "we are modernizing the office. In future all our drawing will be done by computer. You will have to join the other tracers on a course to learn how to do it." Before my illness, I was so stuck in my ways I would have told him to "keep his job", but needs must and I just got on with it. I was lucky to have a job. Bob wasn't taking to redundancy at all well. He hadn't been able to get another job straight away and was getting very depressed. He was frustrated, but it was still a shock when I got a phone call at work to say he had been rushed into hospital with a heart attack. He ended up with a by-pass operation. We really felt that somebody had it in for us. We clung on to the joy we experienced at the birth of our granddaughter; it was this that seemed to make everything worthwhile.

'After all we had been through, Bob and I could count ourselves as survivors; we felt that there was nothing more that could happen that we couldn't handle. Life seemed quite different after that. I don't think I would have looked after myself if Bob hadn't needed some encouragement to go regularly to the leisure centre to exercise to strengthen his heart. I went with him and joined in, and we have been enjoying our visits ever since. We have made a number of new friends who have had similar experiences and we encourage each other. Eventually, Bob got himself a part-time job as a technician in the lab. at the local tech. He likes being with the youngsters. I am still working full time, and in fact I enjoy working with the computer. I keep saying "Fancy me a granny and being able to use all this complicated technology". Bob helps out by doing all the cooking and shopping – in fact he quite enjoys it. He had never cooked until I became ill. Now he is always experimenting and following a lot of the advice about healthy eating which he was given after he left hospital. Funnily enough, in many ways we are probably a lot fitter than we ever were. This pain I get seems to come when I get tired. I don't think I pace myself well enough. I'm a bit of a terrier, and once I get my teeth into a job I don't want to finish until it's done. My doctor says that you are good at helping people to talk about things that are bothering them and getting them to see how they can help themselves, as well as teaching them how to relax and enjoy life.

'So, do you think you can help me?'

# Useful Addresses

The list is not exhaustive, but a letter or phone call to any one of the following should direct you to the most appropriate source of help for you.

BACUP
121/123 Charterhouse Street,
London EC1M 6AA.
Tel: Cancer Information Service: 0171 608 1611
    Freephone outside London: 0800 181 199

British Association for Counselling,
1 Regent Place,
Rugby CV1 2PJ.
Tel: 01788 578328

Cancerlink,
17 Britannia Street,
London WC1X 9JN.
Tel: 0171 833 2451

*and*

9 Castle Terrace,
Edinburgh EH1 2DP.
Tel: 0131 228 5557

Cancer Relief Macmillan Fund,
Anchor House,
15–19 Britten Street,
London SW3 3TZ.
Tel: 0171 351 7811

*and*

9 Castle Terrace,
Edinburgh EH1 2DP.
Tel: 0131 229 3276

Carers' National Association,
29 Chilworth Mews,
London W2 3RG.
Tel: 0171 724 7776

Hospice Information Service,
St Christopher's Hospice,
51–59 Lawrie Park Road,
Sydenham,
London SE26 6DZ.
Tel: 0181 778 9252

Institute for Complementary Medicine,
PO Box 194,
London SE16 1QZ.
Tel: 0171 237 5165

Irish Cancer Society,
5 Northumberland Road,
Dublin 4.
Tel: Dublin: (01) 681855
      Helpline: (01) 681233

Malcolm Sargent Fund for Children,
14 Abingdon Road,
London W8 6AF.
Tel: 0171 937 4548

Marie Curie Cancer Care,
28 Belgrave Square,
London SW1X 8QG.
Tel: 0171 235 3325

Pain Association Scotland,
Cramond House,
Cramond Glebe Road,
Edinburgh EH4 6NS.
Tel: 0131 312 7955
(For people with chronic pain, including cancer pain.)

USEFUL ADDRESSES

Pain Concern (UK),
PO Box 318,
Canterbury,
Kent CT4 5DP.
Tel: 01227 264677

Ulster Cancer Foundation,
40–42 Eglantine Avenue,
Belfast BT9 6DX.
Tel: 01232 663281
    Helpline: 01232 663439

# Further Reading

Gerald G. Jampolsky, *Love is Letting Go of Fear*. USA: Celestial Arts, 1985.

Nira Kfir and Maurice Slevin, *Challenging Cancer: From Chaos to Control*. Tavistock/Routledge, 1991.

Jo Ann Le Maistre, *Beyond Rage*. USA: Alpine Guild, 1993.

Stephanie Matthews Simonton, *The Healing Family*. Bantam Books, 1988.

John Roger and Peter McWilliams, *You Can't Afford the Luxury of a Negative Thought*. Thorsons, 1991.

Dorothy Rowe, *Beyond Fear*. Fontana, 1987.

Neville Shone, *Coping Successfully with Pain*. Sheldon Press, 1992.

Bernie Siegel, *Love, Medicine and Miracles*. Arrow Books, 1989.

Ann Kaiser Stearns, *Living Through Personal Crisis*. Sheldon Press, 1987.

Rosemary Wells, *Helping Chidren Cope with Grief*. Sheldon Press, 1988.

# Index